Management of Urology

Series Editors

Sanchia S. Goonewardene, Princess Alexandra Hospital, Harlow, UK

Raj Persad, North Bristol NHS Trust, Bristol, UK

This series addresses the need for an increase in the quantity of literature focused upon the effects of cancer in urology. Books within it will draw attention to the management of subtype specific urology cancer patients at each step of their pathway with suggestions on how care can potentially be improved. Therefore, it is of interest to a range of trainee and practicing physicians in a range of disciplines including urology oncology, specialist nurse and general practitioners.

Oliver Brunckhorst • Kamran Ahmed
Asif Muneer • Hussain M Alnajjar
Editors

Penile Cancer – A Practical Guide

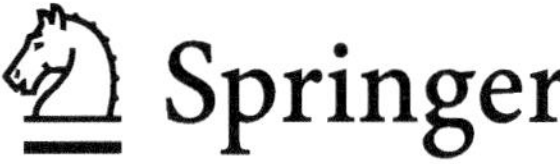

Editors
Oliver Brunckhorst
King's College London
London, UK

Kamran Ahmed
King's College London
London, UK

Asif Muneer
University College London Hospital and
University College London
London, UK

Hussain M Alnajjar
University College London Hospital and
University College London
London, UK

This work contains media enhancements, which are displayed with a "play" icon. Material in the print book can be viewed on a mobile device by downloading the Springer Nature "More Media" app available in the major app stores. The media enhancements in the online version of the work can be accessed directly by authorized users.

ISSN 2730-6372 ISSN 2730-6380 (electronic)
Management of Urology
ISBN 978-3-031-32683-7 ISBN 978-3-031-32681-3 (eBook)
https://doi.org/10.1007/978-3-031-32681-3

This Springer imprint is published by the registered company Springer Nature Switzerland AG
The registered company address is: Gewerbestrasse 11, 6330 Cham, Switzerland

Your bonus with the purchase of this book

With the purchase of this book, you can use our"SN Flashcards" app to access questions free of charge in order to test your learning and check your understanding of the contents of the book.
To use the app, please follow the instructions below:

1. Go to **https://flashcards.springernature.com/login**
2. Create an user account by entering your e-mail adress and assiging a password.
3. Use the link provided in one of the first chapters to access your SN Flashcards set.

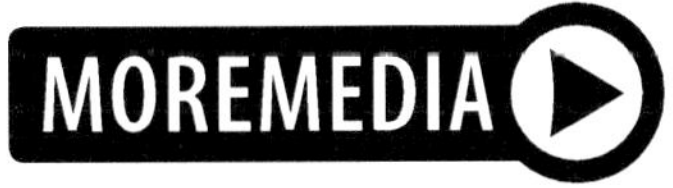

Your personal SN Flashcards link is provided in one of the first chapters.

If the link is missing or does not work, please send an e-mail with the subject "**SN Flashcards**" and the book title to **customerservice@springernature.com**.

Preface

Penile cancer can be a daunting topic for many. The increasing centralization of care into specialist centres combined with the relative rarity of the disease itself means that exposure to the disease can at times be limited. However, an understanding of the disease process and its management remains essential for ensuring healthcare professionals can deliver good care when it is encountered. Furthermore, it remains a commonly covered area in many exit examinations for specialist certification.

However, we found that unfortunately many textbooks on penile cancer are aimed at the supra specialist level, thereby covering the subject area in more detail than necessary for the average healthcare professional and trainee. With this in mind, we decided to produce this textbook *Penile Cancer—a Practical Guide* and is aimed at any healthcare professionals who may encounter penile cancer during their practice. The book promises to be a particularly useful tool for those currently in training, and who are working towards their specialist final examinations.

In this textbook, we provide a more succinct summary of all aspects of penile cancer care. From the aetiology and molecular biology of disease, diagnostic workup of patients to differing surgical or non-surgical management techniques. We have gathered experts from across the globe to cover these topics, providing up-to-date and evidence-based summaries of the required knowledge on the topic. Chapters also come with key points and practice multiple choice and viva style questions to reinforce essential learning points, meaning this textbook can act as a useful learning tool prior to any examinations.

We hope you find this textbook useful and enjoy reading it as much as we have when putting it together.

London, UK Oliver Brunckhorst
London, UK Kamran Ahmed
London, UK Asif Muneer
London, UK Hussain M Alnajjar

Acknowledgements

We would like to express our enormous gratitude to all authors who have contributed to this textbook. Without your invaluable expert knowledge, and most importantly time provided to produce such fantastic chapters, this book would not have been possible. Additionally, we would like to thank Sanchia Goonewardene, Raj Persad, and the production team at Springer for enabling us to produce this textbook within their 'Management of Urology' Series.

Finally, and certainly not least, to all our colleagues, friends, and family whose unwavering patience and support make projects such as these possible.

Contents

1 **Epidemiology and Aetiology of Penile Cancer** 1
Jonathan Cobley and Aditya Manjunath

2 **Pathology and Molecular Biology of Penile Cancer** 13
Aiman Haider and Alex Freeman

3 **Imaging Techniques Used in Penile Cancer** 31
Alex Kirkham and Adam Retter

4 **Diagnosing and Staging Patients with Penile Cancer** 51
Alice Yu, Jad Chahoud, Jasreman Dhillon, and Philippe E. Spiess

5 **Premalignant Penile Lesions** 65
Thomas T. F. Wong, Martin Mak, Hussain M Alnajjar, and Wayne Lam

6 **Penile-Sparing Surgical Options for Patients Diagnosed with Penile Cancer** 83
James A. Churchill and Vijay K. Sangar

7 **Surgical Management of Advanced Penile Cancer** 97
Yao Zhu, Dingwei Ye, and Weijie Gu

8 **How to Manage the Lymph Nodes in Penile Cancer** 109
Giuseppe Fallara, Andrea Salonia, and Asif Muneer

9 **The Role of Chemotherapy and Radiotherapy in Penile Cancer** 127
Constantine Alifrangis and Anita Mitra

10 **Reconstructive Surgical Techniques in Penile Cancer** 137
Laura Elst, Wai Gin Lee, and Maarten Albersen

11 **Late Effects of Penile Cancer** 163
Clare Akers, Stanley Tang, Oliver Brunckhorst, and Matthew Rewhorn

About the Editors

Oliver Brunckhorst, MBBS, BSc (Hons), MRCS (Eng) Having undertaken his medical training at Imperial College London, Oliver graduated with distinctions in Medical Science, Clinical Science, and Clinical Practice and received the Imperial College Faculty of Medicine Prize for his overall final performance. He additionally, undertook an intercalated BSc at King's College London in Anatomy, Developmental and Human Biology graduating with First Class Honours. He subsequently was appointed as a surgical Academic Foundation Doctor at Imperial College London and Northwest Thames Deanery and subsequently as an NIHR Urology Academic Clinical Fellow at King's College London and London South Urology Deanery. Along with his Urology training, he is undertaking a PhD in Urology at King's College London.

His interests in academic urology now primarily include wellbeing and quality of life in men's health and cancer, acting as lead co-ordinator for several studies, including the multi-institutional MIND-P prospective cohort study. In addition to this, he has focussed on surgical education, curriculum development, and the role of non-technical skills in operating theatres. These have resulted in over 50 peer-reviewed journal publications to date in high impact journals, along with numerous national and international meeting presentations which have included several best poster prizes. Additionally, he is co-editor of the book *Men's Health and Wellbeing* and has authored seven book chapters in clinical, education, men's health, and anatomical subjects. Oliver is also a keen educator regularly teaching medical students, as a clinical skills tutor and lecturer on the Surgical Sciences intercalated BSc programme at King's College London.

Kamran Ahmed, MBBS, MRCS, PhD, FRCS Urol Kamran is urologist with a specialist interest in Andrology including male sexual/erectile dysfunction, Peyronie's disease, low testosterone management, male fertility, vasectomy reversal, and urethral stricture surgery (endoscopic and reconstructive). He completed his specialist urology training in London and undertook a clinical fellowship training at the University College London Hospital in Andrology, men's reconstructive surgery, and infertility management.

He holds a PhD degree in Surgical Education from Imperial College London and his research interests include surgical education (curriculum and assessment tools development and validation), men's health and survivorship, sperm retrieval techniques, and management of infertility in non-obstructive azoospermia. He has received several awards, and both clinical and educational grants, from organizations, including the European Association of Urology, the British Association of Urological Surgeons, the Royal College of Surgeons, the National Institute for Health Research, the Coptcoat Charity, and Pelican Group.

Mr Ahmed has published widely, with nearly 300 peer-reviewed indexed publications and around 300 national and international conference presentations. He is editor and author of four urological textbooks and has written several book chapters. His roles include the lead for Surgical Sciences iBSc modules at KCL, education lead for EULIS section of European Association of Urology (EAU), board member of Junior ERUS-EAU, and tutor on the European Urology Resident

Education Programme (EUREP). He has been invited as visiting professor or lecturer to institutions in the USA, Europe, and Middle East. He is currently the Director of IRB (Institutional Review Board) committee at Sheikh Khalifa Medical City, Abu Dhabi. He is the research lead for Sheikh Khalifa Medical City, UAE.

Sheikh Khalifa Medical City, Abu Dhabi, UAE
Khalifa University, Abu Dhabi, UAE
King's College London, London, UK

Asif Muneer, BSc, MB, ChB, FRCS (Urol), MD Professor Asif Muneer MD FRCS(Urol) is Professor of Urology and Surgical Andrology at the University College London. He is also a Consultant Urological Surgeon and Andrologist based at the University College London Hospital, UK. Having completed his higher degree (MD) at the Wolfson Institute, UCL he went on to complete his higher surgical training at the University of Oxford Higher Surgical Training Scheme. He then undertook further visiting fellowships to develop surgical expertise at the University of Bern, University of Paris, The NKI in Amsterdam, and MD Anderson, Texas. He has received a number of national awards including the Intercollegiate Gold Medal for the FRCS(Urol) as well as the Harold Hopkins Golden Telescope from the British Association of Urological Surgeons.

Professor Muneer has published extensively in peer-reviewed journals and has also edited several textbooks including *Viva Practice for the FRCS(Urol)* (1st and 2nd editions), *Textbook of Penile Cancer* (1st and 2nd editions), *Prosthetic Surgery in Urology and Atlas of Male Genitourethral Surgery*. He is a key opinion leader in the field of male genital cancer; he has also developed novel surgical techniques and published extensively in the field of Penile Cancer and leads one of the largest international Penile Cancer Networks and is the Chief Investigator for the National Institute of Health Research VELRAD trial.

University College London Hospitals, London, UK
University College London, London, UK

Hussain M Alnajjar, BSc, MBBS, ChM, FEBU, FRCS(Urol) Hussain Alnajjar is a Consultant Urological Surgeon and Andrologist at the University College London Hospital (UCLH). He is an Honorary Associate Professor at the University College London.

His practice includes managing quaternary referrals; his areas of expertise include Peyronie's disease, penile prosthesis surgery, penile cancer, and male genital reconstruction. He has won several coveted accolades for his clinical and academic achievements. Mr Alnajjar has published widely in a number of high impact factor peer-reviewed medical journals and has written numerous book chapters within the field of Andrology. He remains actively involved in clinical research in his field.

Mr Alnajjar is an avid mentor and a trainer for senior Andrology fellows. He is a member of the European Board of Urology examination committee and an examiner for the membership examination of the Royal College of Surgeons of England.

University College London Hospitals, London, UK
University College London, London, UK

Abbreviations

5-FU	5-fluorouracil
AJCC	American Joint Committee on Cancer
ALT	Anterolateral thigh
BAUS	British Association of Urological Surgeons
BLT	Buschke-Löwenstein tumour
BD	Bowen's disease
BMG	Buccal mucosa graft
BMI	Body mass index
BP	Bowenoid papulosis
CIS	Carcinoma in situ
CSS	Cancer-specific survival
CT	Computerized tomography
DLT	Decongestive lymphatic therapy
DSNB	Dynamic sentinel node biopsy
EAU	European Association of Urology
EQ	Erythroplasia of Queyrat
FDG	^{18}F-fluorodeoxyglucose
FNA	Fine needle aspiration
H&E	Hematoxylin and Eosin
HPV	Human papilloma virus
ICCR	International Collaboration on Cancer Reporting
IHC	Immunohistochemical
ILNs	Inguinal lymph nodes
ILND	Inguinal lymph node dissection
IDC	Indwelling catheter
ISH	In situ hybridization
ISUP	International Society of Urological Pathology
LA	Local anaesthetic
LND	Lymph node dissection
LVI	Lymphovascular invasion
LSc	Lichen sclerosus
LSEA	Lichen sclerosus et atrophicans
MLD	Musculocutaneous latissimus dorsi
MMR	Mismatch repair

MMS	Moh's micrographic surgery
MRI	Magnetic resonance imaging
NCCN	National Comprehensive Cancer Network
NEC	Neuroendocrine carcinomas
OS	Overall survival
OSS	Organ sparing surgery
PCR	Polymerase chain reaction
PeIN	Penile intraepithelial neoplasia
PET	Positron emission tomography
PLN	Pelvic lymph node
PLND	Pelvic lymph node dissection
PNI	Perineural Invasion
PROMs	Patient-reported outcome measures
PUVA	Psoralen and ultraviolet light A
QOL	Quality of life
RFF	Radial Artery Forearm Free
SCC	Squamous cell carcinoma
STSG	Split-thickness skin graft
TFL	Tensor fascia lata
TIP	Paclitaxel + ifosfamide + cisplatin regimen
TMB	Tumour mutational burden
TTP	Time to progression
UCAPP	Urethral centralization after partial penectomy
UICC	Union Internationale Contre le Cancer
US	Ultrasonography
VRAM	Vertical rectus abdominis myocutaneous
WHO	World Health Organization
WLE	Wide local excision

List of Figures

Fig. 1.1 Penile cancer average number of new cases per year and age-specific incidence rates per 100,000 males, United Kingdom, 2015–2017. Credit: Cancer Research UK 2

Fig. 1.2 Incidence of Penile Cancer by T Stage at authors institution between 2018 and 2021 3

Fig. 1.3 Lichen sclerosus, two photographs from the same patient. There is phimosis with associated thickening and pale discolouration of the unhealthy foreskin. The patient underwent circumcision. Medical photographs reproduced with written consent from a patient treated at North Bristol NHS Trust, October 2021 4

Fig. 2.1 (**a**) Haematoxylin and Eosin stain 20X magnification. Differentiated PeIN with surface maturation and marked atypia of the basal and parabasal keratinocytes. (**b**) MIB-1 stain 20X magnification. Overexpression of proliferation marker in the atypical basal and parabasal cells in differentiated PeIN. (**c**) Immunohistochemistry for p53 (20× magnification) can show 'wild type' staining in differentiated PeIN 15

Fig. 2.2 (**a**) Immunohistochemistry for p16. Magnification 20X. No reactivity for p16 in differentiated PeIN. (**b**) Haematoxylin and Eosin stain 10X Magnification. Differentiated PeIN (pleomorphic variant): Marked pleomorphism of the basal and parabasal keratinocytes. There is surface maturation. (**c**) Immunohistochemistry for p53 10X. Differentiated PeIN: Mutant type staining with strong and diffuse overexpression of p53 in basal and parabasal layers. (**d**) Magnification 20X. Immunohistochemistry for MIB-1 overexpression in the atypical basal and parabasal cells of differentiated PeIN 16

Fig. 2.3 (**a**) Haematoxylin and Eosin stain. Magnification 10X. Undifferentiated PeIN basaloid type. Full thickness atypia of the surface squamous epithelium with a monotonous population of basophilic cells. (**b**) Immunohistochemistry for p16 shows 'en-bloc' strong and diffuse reactivity in undifferentiated PeIN 16

Fig. 2.4 Immunohistochemistry for p53. Magnification 4X. p53 overexpression (diffuse and continuous staining) in differentiated PeIN in contrast to the intermittent basal staining seen in the background surface squamous epithelium. 17
Fig. 2.5 (**a**) Hematocylin and Eosin 10X magnification. Typical Condyloma. Benign squamoproliferative lesion with hyperkeratosis, parakeratosis, acanthosis and papillomatosis of the surface squamous epithelium. (**b**) Immunohistochemistry for p16 shows focal/ scattered reactivity for p16 in the surface keratinocytes. (**c**) Haematoxylin and Eosin 10X. Typical condyloma 18
Fig. 2.6 Haemtoxylin and Eosin 40X. Atypical Condyloma. Mild to moderate pleomorphism with frequent mitotic figures 18
Fig. 2.7 (**a**) Haematoxylin and Eosin 4X. Lichen sclerosus. Attenuation and thinning of the surface squamous epithelium with subepithelial sclerosus and vascular ectasia. (**b**) Haematoxylin and Eosin 4X. Lichen sclerosus. Subepithelial sclerosus and a patchy lichenoid chronic inflammatory cell infiltrate 19
Fig. 2.8 Haematoxylin and Eosin 10X. Basaloid squamous cell carcinoma 20
Fig. 2.9 (**a**) Haematoxylin and Eosin stain 10X. Sarcomatoid carcinoma composed of a prominent component of pleomorphic spindle cells in interlacing fascicles. (**b**) Haematoxylin and Eosin stain 10X magnification. An adjacent focus of admixed squamous cell carcinoma helps establish the diagnosis of sarcomatoid carcinoma. 21
Fig. 3.1 Penile anatomy visible on MRI and ultrasound. Axial section at mid shaft. With permission from Muneer A and Horenblas S, *Textbook of Penile Cancer*, Springer International Publishing 33
Fig. 3.2 Axial T2-weighted (**a**, **b**) and T1-weighted (**c**) images through the penis in different patients after intracavernosal alprostadil. Note the differing conspicuity of Buck's fascia and the dorsal vessels: clearly visible in patients (**a**, **c**) but not (**b**). *Black arrowheads* mark the tunica albuginea, and *white arrowheads* Buck's fascia. The *thick white arrow* shows the superficial dorsal vein in (**a**), and the thinner *white arrows* the deep dorsal vessels. The cavernosal arteries are marked by *black arrows*. The urethra, lying in the middle of the corpus spongiosum, is marked by an *asterisk*. Note the layering of signal within the corpora cavernosa in (**b**), a normal finding. With permission from Muneer A and Horenblas S, *Textbook of Penile Cancer*, Springer International Publishing 34
Fig. 3.3 T2-weighted coronal section through the base (**a**) and shaft (**b**) of the penis after intracavernosal alprostadil. In (**a**) a *white arrowhead* marks the ischiocavernosus muscle, and a *black*

arrowhead the bulbocavernosus. A *white arrow* shows the urethra entering the bulb. Inferior pubic rami are marked by *asterisks*. In (**b**), a *black arrowhead* marks the tunica albuginea and a *white arrowhead* Buck's fascia. The glans is well seen (*thick white arrows*). With permission from Muneer A and Horenblas S, *Textbook of Penile Cancer*, Springer International Publishing 35

Fig. 3.4 Two axial images of the shaft of the tumescent penis: the first (**a**) taken at an angle of 45° to avoid diffraction artifact, and the second (**b**), in the standard transverse plane with the probe ventral. The urethra (*white arrow*) is sometimes seen well within the corpus spongiosum. Tunica albuginea and Buck's fascia (*black arrows*) appear as one echogenic layer, thickest around the corpora cavernosa. *White arrowheads* show superficial vessels, and *black arrowheads* the cavernosal vessels. With permission from Muneer A and Horenblas S, *Textbook of Penile Cancer*, Springer International Publishing 35

Fig. 3.5 T2-weighted sagittal section close to the midline (**a**) after intracavernosal alprostadil and (**b**) without tumescence. *Black arrows* mark the tunica albuginea, large *white arrows* the corpus spongiosum, small *white arrows* the urethra within it, and *black arrows* the bulbocavernosus muscle. The *white arrow head* marks the entry of the urethra into the roof of the bulb. An *asterisk* marks the glans. The 'corrugated' appearance of the corpus cavernosum in (**a**) is because of the midline intercavernosal septum. Note the considerably thicker tunica albuginea in the detumescent state, and the lower signal in the corpus cavernosum; the glans is not in the midline sagittal plane. With permission from Muneer A and Horenblas S, *Textbook of Penile Cancer*, Springer International Publishing 37

Fig. 3.6 Ulcerating lesion on the glans (*white arrowheads*, with a *white arrow* showing the ulcerated part), pT2 on histology and correctly called T2 on MRI (**a**) and ultrasound (**b**). CC marks corpus cavernosum, and S the spongiosal part of the glans. Note that on MR the underlying high signal of the spongiosal tissue of the glans is altered by the tumour, although the tips of the cavernosa are well seen and not involved. The ultrasound confirms involvement of the spongiosal tissue of the glans but not the corpora cavernosa. With permission from Muneer A and Horenblas S, Textbook of Penile Cancer, Springer International Publishing. 38

Fig. 3.7 While most T3 tumours may be adequately assessed clinically, and excision margins confirmed by frozen section, imaging helps to show these rare cases of a skip lesion in the corpus cavernosum. In (**a**), two discrete tumour foci are seen in the corpora cavernosa on T2-weighted MRI (confirmed as discontinuous on histology). In a Doppler ultrasound image from another patient (**b**), a hypervascular nodule (*white arrows*) is seen discrete from the main tumour mass (*arrowheads*). A *black arrow* marks the normal cavernosal artery. With permission from Muneer A and Horenblas S, *Textbook of Penile Cancer*, Springer International Publishing 39

Fig. 3.8 (**a–c**) Features of a benign lymph node (*arrowheads*) on ultrasound, doppler ultrasound, and MRI respectively. Note the fatty hila in each case (*white arrow*). The ultrasound shows ovoid nodes with a regular cortex of uniform thickness; on doppler (**b**), small vessels radiate symmetrically from the hilum (*small white arrows*). MRI (**c**) shows nodes in *short axis*: approximately round, but with fatty hila and regular cortex. With permission from Muneer A and Horenblas S, *Textbook of Penile Cancer*, Springer International Publishing 40

Fig. 3.9 Several features of malignant nodes. (**a**) Ultrasound shows an enlarged node with eccentric, lobulated enlargement of the cortex (*arrowheads* show the hilum, and the *arrows* the eccentric widening), and (**b**) a doppler trace of the same node showing a resistive index of 1.2. (**c–f**) Malignant nodes (*arrowheads*) with necrosis on ultrasound, CT, T2-weighted MRI, and postcontrast MRI (in different patients). The necrotic focus (*white arrow*, (**c**)) is nearly anechoic on ultrasound. On CT (**d**) it is of low density (close to water). (**e**) A node consisting of an eccentric nodule (*black arrow*) and fluid necrosis (*white arrow*) on a T2-weighted axial MR sequence. (**f**) A postcontrast gradient echo fat-saturated coronal sequence of the same node showing the non-enhancing necrotic component. With permission from Muneer A and Horenblas S, *Textbook of Penile Cancer*, Springer International Publishing 41

Fig. 3.10 (**a**) Thick-slab T1 spin echo coronal image of the superficial inguinal nodes. The horizontal group is shown by the *white arrows*: the most medial (*asterisk*) is defined as the 'sentinel' node. *Black arrowheads* mark the superficial epigastric vein; note that on the left the sentinel node lies medial to the superficial epigastric vein, but on the right is anterior to it. *White arrowheads* mark the long saphenous vein and the *black arrow* the junction between the superficial epigastric and long saphenous veins. (**b**) Axial T2-weighted image of the groin in a patient scanned because of a penile prosthesis. Note the horizontal chain of the superficial nodes (*small white arrows*, each with a fatty hilum). They lie superficial to the fascia lata (*white arrowheads*). The saphenous vein (*black arrow*) passes through the cribriform fascia (lying in the oval defect of the fascia lata) to join the femoral vein (*v*). The femoral artery is marked a, the femoral nerve *n*, and the spermatic cord *s*. The *larger white arrow* shows a deep inguinal node medial to the femoral vein. With permission from Muneer A and Horenblas S, *Textbook of Penile Cancer*, Springer International Publishing . . . 44

Fig. 4.1 Penile squamous cell carcinoma, flat lesion, affecting the meatus . . . 52

Fig. 4.2 Summary of metastatic work up for penile cancer . . . 56

Fig. 5.1 Penile intraepithelial neoplasia (PeIN) of the glans and inner foreskin . . . 67

Fig. 5.2 Total glans resurfacing for a patient with PeIN. (**a**) 4 quadrants marker done with the meatus marked separately; (**b**, **c**): Individual quadrants are excised carefully by dissecting the epithelial and subepithelial layers (**d**) The denuded glans with a spatulated neomeatus . . . 74

Fig. 5.3 Mounting of specimen mounted on a plastic surface to assist with more accurate pathological assessment. A separate meatal margin was also taken . . . 75

Fig. 5.4 Split thickness graft post excision. (**a**) Split thickness graft is applied onto the denuded spongy tissue of the glans; (**b**) The neoglans with a split thickness skin graft and quilted sutures to allow graft take . . . 75

Fig. 6.1 Surgical procedure options by tumour location and T-stage . . . 85

Fig. 6.2 Penile squamous cell carcinoma. Image courtesy of Mr. Arie Parnham . . . 94

Fig. 7.1 Flow chart for management of advanced penile cancer. *FNA* fine-needle aspiration, *DSNB* dynamic sentinel node biopsy, *LND* lymph node dissection . . . 98

Fig. 7.2 Case 1 (**a**) Fixed and ulcerated metastatic lymph node (**b**) Complete incision of tumour and overlying skin and subcutaneous tissue (**c**) Mobilization of surrounding abdominal flap to cover the skin defect . . . 101

Fig. 7.3 Case 2 Primary closure of the defect using VRAM flaps (**a**) Widespread invasion of the abdominal and groin skin (**b**) Complete removal of tumours (**c**) Closure of the abdominal and groin wound . . . 102

Fig. 8.1 Left bulging mass after glansectomy and right radical inguinal lymph node dissection for cT2N2M0 penile cancer on the glans. The inguinal mass was mobile, dull, not painful. Left radical inguinal lymph node dissection was performed which confirmed the presence of nodal metastasis of penile cancer . . . 112

Fig. 8.2 Example of left dynamic sentinel node biopsy, after wide local excision of penile cancer of the glans (cT1N0M0). The 99mTechnectium-labelled nanocolloid radiotracer is injected in the morning and lymphoscintigraphic images are taken at 0, 10, 20 and 30 min after injection while a SPECT-CT is performed 2 h after the injection. Patent blue dye is injected just before surgery. During surgery a gamma probe, together with palpation and direct visualisation of the patent blue dye, are used to identify the sentinel lymph node(s) 115

Fig. 8.3 Lymphoedema of the scrotum is a possible complication of ILND with an incidence of 50-60% of cases. Surgical indications are mainly for patient discomfort, and bulky lymphoedema. 116

Fig. 8.4 (**a**) Example of radical inguinal lymph node dissection. Skin incision is performed almost 2 cm below the inguinal ligament and dissection is conducted above and below the fascia lata. (**b**) Example of superficial inguinal lymph node dissection. Skin incision is always performed almost 2 cm below the inguinal ligament, shorter than in the case of radical ILND, and dissection is performed above the fascia lata 117

Fig. 10.1 The glans epithelium and subepithelium of each quadrant are dissected from the meatus to the coronal sulcus to remove the tumour 141

Fig. 10.2 (**a**, **b**) An air-powered dermatome is used to harvest the STSG from the thigh. The STSG is used to cover the spongious tissue of the glans. 141

Fig. 10.3 The extragenital STSG is applied over the corpora and the neoglans is quilted with monofilament 5.0 sutures, which compresses the graft to its bed and reduces potential space for hematoma formation 141

Fig. 10.4 Small cuts in the graft are made with the tip of a no. 15 blade in order to evacuate the hematoma under the graft. 142

Fig. 10.5 Appearance of a STSG after application and quilting 143

Fig. 10.6 (**a**) Tie-over dressing to compress the graft against the graft bed (**b**) Tie-over dressing consisting of silicone gauze and multiple layers of paraffin gauze. 143

Fig. 10.7 (**a**) Appearance of STSG after removal of the tie-over dressing one-week post-operative. (**b**) Appearance of STSG 3 months post-operative. 144

Fig. 10.8 (**a**) Example of partial failure of STSG. This lesion will heal spontaneously by granulation of tissue. (**b**) Example of subtotal failure of STSG, due to the avascular graft bed or infection after a glansectomy 144

Fig. 10.9 Subcoronal skin incision. In uncircumcised men a circumcision is performed. 145

Fig. 10.10 Dissection over Buck's fascia. A thorough haemostasis is achieved by bipolar diathermy. 146
Fig. 10.11 The dissection continues until the entire glans is dissected of the corporal heads and only the urethra remains intact. Finally, the urethra is transected and placed within the corpora cavernosa 146
Fig. 10.12 (**a, b**) The urethra is spatulated and fixed to the corpora. Afterwards the penile shaft skin is sutured to the tunica albuginea of the underlying corporal bodies with 4.0 polyglactin sutures, forming a neoglans 146
Fig. 10.13 Dissection under Buck's fascia with identification of the neurovascular bundle 147
Fig. 10.14 The buccal mucosa graft is indicated and stretched with stay sutures. Hydrodissection is achieved by means of infiltration with Lidocaine hydrochloride 1% and with epinephrine 1:100,000 to enhance haemostasis of the donor site 149
Fig. 10.15 The BMG is carefully defatted and prepared 150
Fig. 10.16 The graft is sewn into the glans cleft with the mucosal part facing the lumen 151
Fig. 10.17 Appearance of a buccal mucosa inlay without closure, one-year post-operative 151
Fig. 10.18 Single cylinder device prepared with Dacron cap in place. 155
Fig. 10.19 The neophallus deflated 156
Fig. 10.20 The neophallus inflated. 156
Fig. 11.1 (**a**, **b**) Meatal Stenosis with Lichen Sclerosus and Penile Carcinoma in Situ (**c**, **d**) Meatal Stenosis After Glans Resurfacing 164
Fig. 11.2 Penile lymphoedema with lymphangioma circumscriptum (arrow) (Images courtesy of Mr. Hussain Alnajjar, UCLH) 166
Fig. 11.3 Batman Technique for genital lymphoedema (Images courtesy of Mr. Hussain Alnajjar, UCLH) 167
Fig. 11.4 Components of wellbeing in penile cancer 168

List of Tables

Table 2.1 WHO Classification of PeIN 14
Table 2.2 2022 World Health Organization classification of invasive epithelial tumours of the penis and scrotum 20
Table 2.3 ICCR carcinoma of the penis dataset 23
Table 2.4 Percentage frequency of somatic mutations in penile SCC 23
Table 3.1 Additional sequences used in MRI. 36
Table 4.1 Differential diagnosis of penile lesion 53
Table 4.2 The AJCC TNM (tumour, node, and metastasis) staging system for penile cancer, 8th ed., 2017 54
Table 4.3 AJCC anatomic stage/prognostic groups 54
Table 5.1 Examples of HPV related and non-HPV related premailignant penile lesions 66
Table 7.1 The presentation of advanced penile cancer. 98
Table 7.2 Preoperative assessment 99
Table 9.1 Side effects of commonly utilised chemotherapy agents 128
Table 9.2 Summary of European Association of Urology Guidelines for chemotherapy in patients with penile cancer 130
Table 9.3 Common side effects of penile brachytherapy 132
Table 10.1 Indications and Surgical Options for Penile Sparing Treatments by Stage of Disease. European Association of Urology (EAU) guidelines on penile cancer, National Comprehensive Cancer Network (NCCN) guidelines on penile cancer 139
Table 11.1 Examples of psychometric tools to evaluate mental wellbeing . . . 170

1 Epidemiology and Aetiology of Penile Cancer

Jonathan Cobley and Aditya Manjunath

Learning Objectives

After reading this chapter you will be able to:

- Define penile cancer incidence and its variation globally and across age groups
- Outline the incidence of penile cancer according to stage at presentation
- Describe the aetiology of penile cancer including both modifiable and non-modifiable risk factors

Introduction

Penile cancer is a rare urological malignancy presenting most commonly in men in their sixth and seventh decades of life [1]. Squamous cell carcinoma accounts for greater than 95% of cases and most commonly affects the glans, coronal sulcus and inner prepuce – essentially the mucosal surfaces. There are several recognised risk factors including phimosis, lack of circumcision, Human Papillomavirus (HPV) infection, lichen sclerosus, poor hygiene, smoking, obesity, immunodeficiency, chronic inflammation, Psoralen and Ultraviolet light A (PUVA) exposure.

J. Cobley · A. Manjunath (✉)
North Bristol NHS Trust, Bristol, UK
e-mail: aditya.m@doctors.org.uk

O. Brunckhorst et al. (eds.), *Penile Cancer – A Practical Guide*, Management of Urology, https://doi.org/10.1007/978-3-031-32681-3_1

Epidemiology

There is substantial global geographical variations in penile cancer incidence. The USA and Europe have a lower incidence than South America, Africa, and Asia. The lowest reported incidence is 0.1 cases per 100,000 in Israel, a country with a near 100% rate of neonatal circumcision and a strong public healthcare system [2]. In comparison, Brazil has the highest reported incidence worldwide at between 2.8 and 6.8 per 100,000 [3].

The global geographical disparity of countries with higher incidence is thought to be secondary to poor socioeconomic status and lower rates of neonatal circumcision [4]. This is further supported by evidence of notable regional differences within countries. In terms of overall relative incidence, penile cancer accounted for 2.1% of male cancers in Brazil, reaching 5.7% in the Northeast region compared to 1.2% in the Southern region [3]. Penile cancer was noted to predominantly affect white, uncircumcised males from low-income areas.

The incidence of penile cancer in the United Kingdom (UK) is between 1.5 to 2.5 per 100,000 men [5]. Significant regional variation exists with areas of greater socio-economic deprivation suffering the highest incidence. From 2013–2017 in England, incidence rates in males were 52% higher in the most deprived quintile compared with the least. In the UK, penile cancer care is centralised into supra-regional networks treating a minimum population size of four million [6]. Centralisation of this rare malignancy has shown to improve survival and have better functional outcomes, with higher use of organ-sparing treatments and invasive inguinal lymph node staging [7, 8].

Penile cancer incidence increases with age (Fig. 1.1). The peak incidence appears to be in men aged 65–69. There is also an increase in the number of younger men

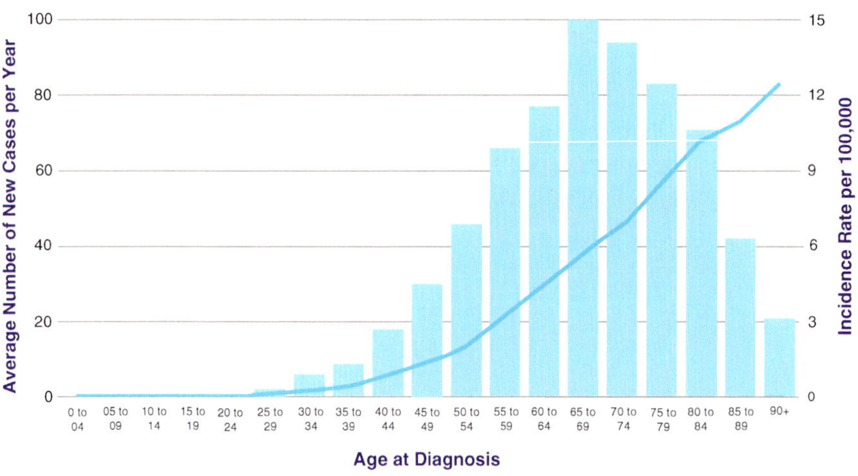

Fig. 1.1 Penile cancer average number of new cases per year and age-specific incidence rates per 100,000 males, United Kingdom, 2015–2017. Credit: Cancer Research UK [5]

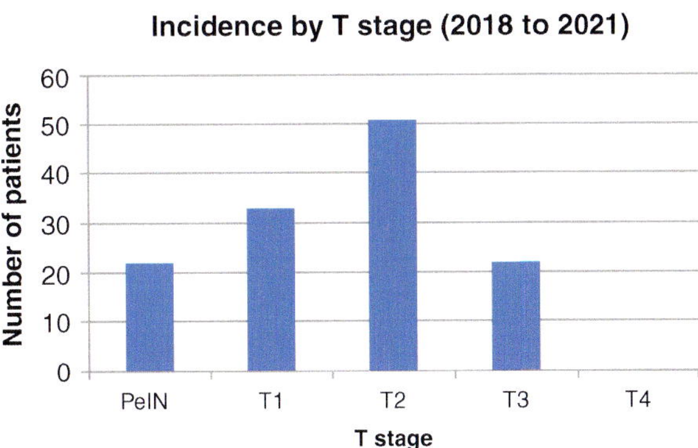

Fig. 1.2 Incidence of Penile Cancer by T Stage at authors institution between 2018 and 2021 [12]

presenting with invasive penile cancer and pre-malignant change. This is thought to be due to the higher prevalence of HPV infection in this cohort. In some countries gender neutral HPV vaccination programmes have commenced to include pre-pubertal boys. In the UK from July 2018 the HPV vaccine has been offered to boys aged 12–13 years [9]. A large cross-sectional study in one of the highest volume centres for penile cancer treatment in Northern Brazil, managed 378 patients with penile cancer over a ten-year period. The age ranged from 25–91 years, whilst cellular features of HPV were identified in 76% of the cohort; it had no impact on prognosis [10].

Presentation by T Stage

Penile cancer is staged using the TNM staging system [11]. The authors unpublished data [12] presented below shows incidence by T stage (Fig. 1.2).

This shows that most patients present with stage T2 disease which is routinely managed by organ sparing surgery. Penile intraepithelial neoplasia (PeIN) refers to carcinoma in situ and in our series accounts for just over 20% of cases.

Aetiology

Most penile cancers are squamous cell carcinomas. The individual risk factors are discussed in more detail in this section.

Phimosis and Inflammatory Conditions Including Lichen Sclerosus

Phimosis is the inability to retract the foreskin and is one of the most important risk factors for developing invasive penile cancer [13]. Neonatal circumcision eliminates the risk of developing pathological phimosis in later life and reports of patients who were circumcised as children developing penile cancer are extremely rare [14].

Lichen Sclerosus (LS) is a chronic inflammatory condition which commonly affects the anogenital region of men and women. LSc causes chronic inflammation of the foreskin and glans penis (Fig. 1.3). Although topical steroids can be used to treat LS, refractory cases can lead to phimosis and urethral stricture disease. The association between LS and vulval cancer is well established but its role in the development of penile cancer is less clear [15]. Oxidative stress can cause DNA damage and lipid peroxidation which is also associated with mutations in tumour suppressor genes [16]. An observational study by Barbagli [17] reviewed the histology of 130 male patients with genital lichen sclerosus over a ten-year period. They found that 11 men (8.4%) had pre-malignant or malignant changes with a mean time between presentation with LS and diagnosis of cancer of 12 years.

Inflammation and/or penile trauma can be a precursor to tumour growth. Both posthitis and balanitis are more prevalent in patients who go on to develop penile cancer [18, 19].

Chronic inflammation is thought to play a role in the development of multiple different cancer subtypes and sites [20]. The production of reactive oxygen and nitrogen species by inflammatory cells have been implicated in the development of numerous different cancer types [21]. The exact mechanisms involved in penile cancer are poorly understood. They may be divided into HPV-dependent or HPV-independent pathways [22]. The latter seems to be affected more frequently by gene alterations. Damage to the p16 tumour suppressor gene has been frequently observed in penile cancer and is discussed in greater detail in Chap. 2 of this book. Adult circumcision is the treatment of choice to manage pathological phimosis and treat chronic inflammation. However, whilst this does reduce the risk of penile cancer development as there is no foreskin, this risk is not reduced to zero.

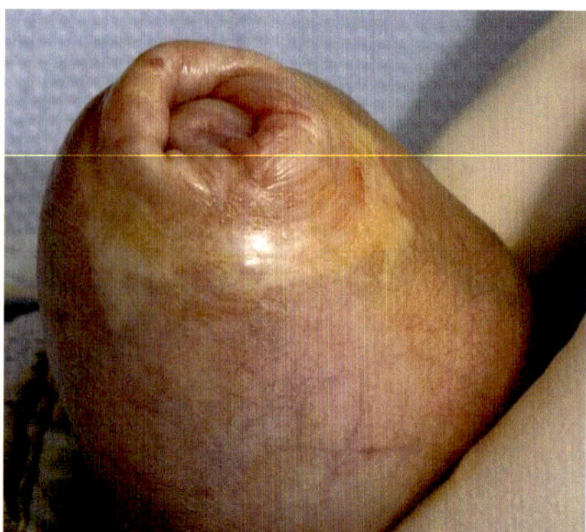
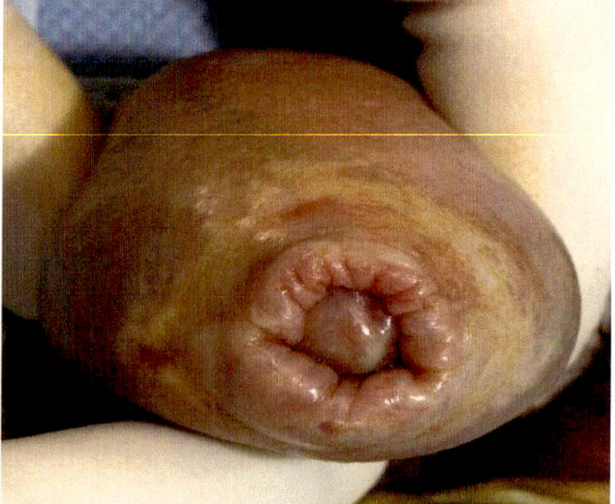

Fig. 1.3 Lichen sclerosus, two photographs from the same patient. There is phimosis with associated thickening and pale discolouration of the unhealthy foreskin. The patient underwent circumcision. Medical photographs reproduced with written consent from a patient treated at North Bristol NHS Trust, October 2021

Circumcision and its Protective Effect

Circumcision in childhood significantly reduces the risk of invasive penile cancer but circumcision does not appear to influence the risk of developing pre-malignant change, irrespective of the age when performed [23]. The protective effect of circumcision is thought to be due to resultant improved hygiene, prevention of smegma build up, lower risk of balanoposthitis and reduced transmission of HPV and HIV [24]. However, adult circumcision has an uncertain or unproven protective role with mixed evidence. Whilst one historical study even associated it with an increased risk of invasive penile cancer [25], this may not demonstrate true causality because the indication for circumcision (for example phimosis or recurrent balanoposthitis) may have been a key factor in the development of subsequent penile cancer. In addition, circumcision may reveal abnormalities which could not be examined before surgery, or it may have been performed as a treatment modality for penile cancer confined to the foreskin [13].

Obesity and Hygiene

Obesity is an increasingly prevalent condition in many countries and has been clearly linked to increased incidence of 13 types of cancer, accounting for a population attributable factor of 3.6% [26]. Since 1980, the prevalence of obesity has doubled in more than 70 countries [27]. Evidence linking obesity directly to penile cancer remains limited, perhaps due to its rarity, but a recent study reported a 53% increased risk of invasive penile cancer for every five-unit increase in Body Mass Index (BMI) [28].

The relationship between obesity and the development of malignant cells is multifactorial and the biological mechanisms are not yet fully understood but adipose tissue is a rich source of endocrine and metabolic activity. A state of hyperinsulinaemia and its cellular growth-promoting effects, as well as a chronic inflammatory response seen with obesity are both thought to be important factors [29] in carcinogenesis.

Obesity is a risk factor for diabetes which has been linked with increased incidence of phimosis [30]. An increased body-mass index is the most common cause for adults who develop a buried penis [31]. This can in turn lead to difficulty maintaining personal hygiene and chronic inflammation of the penis [32]. LS may result from or be a causative factor in the acquisition of a buried penis [33], whilst self-examination is more difficult and may result in delayed presentation.

Given the association between inflammation and penile cancer, it seems logical that poor hygiene could predispose patients to a higher risk of inflammatory conditions. One Danish study [34] reported a falling incidence of penile cancer across a 47-year period which coincided with an increased proportion of Danish accommodation having a bath, rising from 35% in 1940 to 90% in 1990. There was no simultaneous change in national circumcision rates and the authors postulated that this drop in incidence could be related to improved hygiene standards.

Human Papillomavirus (HPV) and Penile Cancer

It is well recognised that HPV, in particular HPV subtypes 16 and 18 play a role in the development of squamous cell cancers [35]. These include oropharyngeal, anal, cervical, and penile cancers. The prevalence of HPV in men is estimated to be greater than 20% in most studies looking at this, although there is large variation geographically. In high-risk groups the prevalence has been reported to be as high as 93% [36]. In most people, the immune system clears the virus from the body by 12 months and no disease occurs. In routine clinical practice, assessment of the presence of HPV itself is difficult to determine therefore a surrogate marker, p16, is used.

Tissue analysed from men with pre-malignant penile lesions (PeIN) and invasive SCCs found that HPV was present in 70–100% of premalignant lesions and 30–40% of invasive tumours [37]. HPV is not implicated in all penile cancer subtypes; it is much more common in warty and basaloid subtypes. It is estimated that 33–66% of warty/basaloid penile cancers contain HPV DNA.

HPV DNA transcribes oncogenes E5, E6 and E7. E6 and E7 viral oncogenes are implicated in malignant transformation of the infected cells. The oncoprotein produced from E6 and E7 genes target the p53 and retinoblastoma-1 (RB1) tumour suppressor genes [38]. Additionally, the oncoprotein E7 produced by high-risk HPV subtypes (16 and 18) binds preferentially to the Rb tumour suppressor protein and leads to over expression of p16. The result is that cell proliferation can proceed uninhibited leading to cancer development.

The prognostic implications of HPV related penile cancers is highly debated. Several studies have reported no difference in lymph node metastases and survival between HPV and non-HPV related tumours; Bezerra et al. [39] found a 68.4% vs 69.1% ten-year survival in the two groups. This contrasts to the findings in a large European study that found a statistically significant 5-year survival benefit in HPV related cancers vs non-HPV - 78% vs 93%, [40].

Although HPV is transmitted by skin to skin contact usually during sexual activity there is no evidence to support a link between penile cancer in men and cervical cancer in their female partners. In the UK females aged 12–13 are routinely offered the HPV vaccine. As mentioned previously this is now also being offered to similar age males. However, the impact this will have on penile cancer incidence will not be known for some time.

Smoking and Tobacco Use

Tobacco use and cigarette smoking has long been a recognised risk factor for developing cancer and was believed to be responsible for 15% of all malignancies in the UK in 2015 [41]. Smoking has been shown to confer between a 2.2–five-fold increased risk of developing penile cancer [42]. The role of smoking in penile cancer is less well documented than in other more common cancers however smoking has been shown to play an important role in histologically similar squamous cancers of the lung and cervix [43]. Daling et al. [44] found that the risks of anogenital cancer increased in proportion to the numbers of cigarettes smoked. Harish and Ravi [45] observed a dose-relationship response for smoking or chewing tobacco and the combination of the two confers a higher risk than smoking or chewing tobacco alone.

Psoralen UV-A Phototherapy (PUVA)

Psoralen is a photosensitizing drug and, given in combination with ultraviolet A, was established as an effective treatment for Psoriasis in 1977. It has since been discovered that a dose-related increased risk of SCC is the most common potential long-term adverse effect of PUVA therapy [46]. In a 12-year study of 892 men undergoing treatment with PUVA, the patients exposed to high levels of PUVA had an incidence of penile invasive squamous-cell carcinoma 286 times that of the general population [47]. A systematic review by Archier et al. [48] found that the risk of SCC increased linearly with the number of treatment sessions and the risk did not reduce on cessation of treatment. The carcinogenic mechanism is not fully understood but is not completely reliant on direct skin exposure to UVA - tumours also occurred on non-exposed penile skin. Patients undergoing treatment therefore require genital protection from PUVA or other UV radiation and genital examination is a critical part of their follow-up.

Key Points

- Penile cancer incidence is highest between the sixth and seventh decades of life, although the incidence seems to be increasing in younger men due to HPV infection
- There is a disparity in incidence of penile cancer both globally and regionally within countries, largely due to socioeconomic inequalities and differences in neonatal circumcision rates
- Squamous cell carcinoma accounts for over 95% of penile cancer cases
- Phimosis is the most important risk factor for developing penile cancer, however circumcision as an adult does not confer protection
- Other risk factors include lichen sclerosus, smoking, HPV, obesity, poor hygiene and exposure to PUVA

Revisions Questions

Multiple Choice Questions

1. Of the following countries, which has the highest incidence of penile cancer?
   A. Thailand
   B. Israel
   C. South Africa
   D. Brazil
   E. Chile

2. Of the following countries, which has the lowest incidence of penile cancer?
   A. Thailand
   B. Israel
   C. South Africa
   D. Brazil
   E. Chile
3. Which of the following strategies would NOT be protective against developing penile cancer?
   A. Smoking cessation
   B. Circumcision aged >18
   C. Neonatal circumcision
   D. Avoiding sexual promiscuity
   E. Regular genital hygiene
4. *Which of the following is NOT a recognised risk factor for developing penile cancer?*
   A. Penile trauma
   B. PUVA treatment for psoriasis
   C. Chewing tobacco
   D. Recurrent balanitis
   E. Marijuana use

Viva Cases

Case 1

A 61-year-old man is referred to see you in clinic with a suspicious marble-sized lump in his glans penis. It has been present for 3 months and has not responded to topical steroids, but his wife is concerned as it has started bleeding.

A. What are the key points to establish from the history?

Case 2

A 31-year-old man is seen in the outpatient clinic asking to be circumcised as his father was diagnosed with penile cancer. He wishes to know if there are any factors that may reduce his own risk of developing the disease

A. What would you advise him?

Answers

Multiple Choice Questions

1. **D.** Brazil has the highest reported incidence worldwide with between 2.8 and 6.8 per 100,000.

2. **B**. Israel has the lowest reported incidence of 0.1 cases per 100,000, thought to be due to a high rate of neonatal circumcision and a strong public health system
3. **B.** Adult circumcision does not have a protective effect against developing penile cancer.
4. **E.** Smoking is a risk factor, but marijuana has not been specifically implicated.

Viva Cases

Case 1

A. The key points to establish from the medical history include:
   - Specific questions about the lump including any change in size, associated pain, bleeding or discharge
   - Does he have a history of phimosis or recurrent inflammation of the foreskin
   - Has he been circumcised, and if so, what age was this performed?
   - Smoking history
   - Sexual history including number of partners
   - Any history of penile trauma
   - Exposure to UV radiation

Case 2

A. Important advice points to cover in the consultation include:
   - Adult circumcision has not been shown to have a protective effect against penile cancer
   - Practice daily genital hygiene and cleanliness
   - Avoid smoking and maintain a healthy weight
   - HPV is transmitted through sexual contact and HPV is also associated with penile cancer. Avoiding sexual promiscuity may be of benefit
   - Regular self-examination should be performed, particularly with a positive family history. Early presentation to general practitioner if any abnormality detected

Test your learning and check your understanding of this book's contents: use the "Springer Nature Flashcards" app to access questions.

To use the app, please follow the instructions below:

1. Go to https://flashcards.springernature.com/login
2. Create a user account by entering your e-mail address and assigning a password
3. Use the following link to access your SN Flashcards set: ▶ https://sn.pub/1r7Om8

If the link is missing or does not work, please send an e-mail with the subject "SN Flashcards" and the book title to customerservice@springernature.com

References

1. Pow-Sang MR, Ferreira U, Pow-Sang JM, Nardi AC, Destefano V. Epidemiology and natural history of penile cancer. Urology. 2010;76(2 Suppl 1):S2-6.
2. Ben Chaim J, Livne PM, Binyamini J, Hardak B, Ben-Meir D, Mor Y. Complications of circumcision in Israel: a one year multicenter survey. Isr Med Assoc J. 2005;7(6):368–70.
3. Favorito LA, Nardi AC, Ronalsa M, et al. Epidemiologic study on penile cancer in Brazil. Int Braz J Urol. 2008;34:587–91. discussion 591-3
4. Douglawi A, Masterson TA. Updates on the epidemiology and risk factors for penile cancer. Transl Androl Urol. 2017;6(5):785–90.
5. Cancer research UK. Penile cancer incidence statistics 2016–2018. Retrieved from: https://www.cancerresearchuk.org/health-professional/cancer-statistics/statistics-by-cancer-type/penile-cancer/incidence Accessed 10/10/2021.
6. Kumar P, Singh S, Goddard JC, Terry TR, Summerton DJ. The development of a supraregional network for the management of penile cancer. Ann R Coll Surg Engl. 2012;94(3):204–9.
7. Quhal F, Pradere B, Mori K, Shariat SF. Volume outcome relationship in penile cancer: a systematic review. Curr Opin Urol. 2020;30(5):696–700.
8. Vanthoor J, Thomas A, Tsaur I, Albersen M, and in collaboration with the European Reference Network for rare urogenital diseases and complex conditions (eUROGEN). Making surgery safer by centralization of care: impact of case load in penile cancer. World J Urol. 2020;38(6):1385–90.
9. Joint Committee on Vaccination and Immunisation Scientific Secretariat. Statement on HPV vaccination. Published July 2020. Retrieved from: https://assets.publishing.service.gov.uk/government/uploads/system/uploads/attachment_data/file/726319/JCVI_Statement_on_HPV_vaccination_2018.pdf Accessed 01/09/2021.
10. Paiva GR, De Oliveira Araújo IB, Athanazio DA, De Freitas LA. Penile cancer: impact of age at diagnosis on morphology and prognosis. Int Urol Nephrol. 2015;47(2):295–9.
11. The American Joint Committee on Cancer. AJCC cancer staging manual. 8th ed. Springer; 2017.
12. Manjunath A, Dickerson D. Data from North Bristol NHS Trust, April 2018–September 2021.
13. Daling JR, et al. Penile cancer: importance of circumcision, human papillomavirus and smoking in in situ and invasive disease. Int J Cancer. 2005;116(4):606–16.
14. Wolbarst AL. Circumcision and penile cancer. Lancet. 1932;1:150–3.
15. Kantere D, Löwhagen GB, Alvengren G, Månesköld A, Gillstedt M, Tunbäck P. The clinical spectrum of lichen sclerosus in male patients—a retrospective study. Acta Derm Venereol. 2014;94(5):542–6.
16. Paulis G, Berardesca E. Lichen sclerosus: the role of oxidative stress in the pathogenesis of the disease and its possible transformation into carcinoma. Res Rep Urol. 2019;11:223–32.
17. Barbagli G, Palminteri E, Mirri F, Guazzoni G, Turini D, Lazzeri M. Penile carcinoma in patients with genital lichen sclerosus: a multicenter survey. J Urol. 2006;175(4):1359–63.
18. Morris BJ, Gray RH, Castellsague X, et al. The strong protective effect of circumcision against cancer of the penis. Adv Urol. 2011;812368
19. Minhas S, Manseck A, Watya S, Hegarty P. Penile cancer—prevention and premalignant conditions. Urology. 2010;76:S24-35.
20. Singh N, Baby D, Rajguru JP, Patil PB, Thakkannavar SS, Pujari VB. Inflammation and cancer. Ann Afr Med. 2019;18(3):121–6.
21. Kruk J, Aboul-Enein HY. Reactive oxygen and nitrogen species in carcinogenesis: implications of oxidative stress on the progression and development of several cancer types. Mini Rev Med Chem. 2017;17:904–19.
22. Chipollini J, Chaing S, Azizi M, Kidd LC, Kim P, Spiess PE. Advances in understanding of penile carcinogenesis: the search for actionable targets. Int J Mol Sci. 2017;18(8):1777.

23. Larke NL, Thomas SL, Dos Santos SI, Weiss HA. Male circumcision and penile cancer: a systematic review and meta-analysis. Cancer Causes Control. 2011;22(8):1097–110.
24. Christodoulidou M, Sahdev V, Houssein S, Muneer A. Epidemiology of penile cancer. Curr Probl Cancer. 2015;39:126–36.
25. Brinton LA, Li JY, Rong SD, Huang S, Xiao BS, Shi BG, et al. Risk factors for penile cancer: results from a case-control study in China. Int J Cancer. 47:504–9.
26. Arnold M, Pandeya N, Byrnes G, Renehan PAG, Stevens GA, Ezzati PM, et al. Global burden of cancer attributable to high body-mass index in 2012: a population-based study. Lancet Oncol. 2015;16(1):36–46.
27. The Global Burden of Disease 2015 Obesity Collaborators. Health effects of overweight and obesity in 195 countries over 25 years. N Engl J Med. 2017;377(1):13–27.
28. Barnes KT, McDowell BD, Button A, Smith BJ, Lynch CF, Gupta A. Obesity is associated with increased risk of invasive penile cancer. BMC Urol. 2016;16(1):42.
29. Renehan AG, Roberts DL, Dive C. Obesity and cancer: pathophysiological and biological mechanisms. Arch Physiol Biochem. 2008;114(1):71–83.
30. Bromage SJ, Crump A, Pearce I. Phimosis as a presenting feature of diabetes. BJU Int. 2008;101(3):338–40.
31. Cohen PR. Adult acquired buried penis: a hidden problem in obese men. Cureus. 2021;13(2):e13067.
32. Smith-Harrison LI, Piotrowski J, Machen GL, Guise A. Acquired buried penis in adults: a review of surgical management. Sex Med Rev. 2020;8(1):150–7.
33. Ho TS, Gelman J. Evaluation and management of adult acquired buried penis. Transl Androl Urol. 2018;7(4):618–27.
34. Frisch M, Friis S, Kjaer SK, Melbye M. Falling incidence of penis cancer in an uncircumcised population (Denmark 1943-90). BMJ. 1995;311(7018):1471.
35. Lebelo RL, Boulet G, Nkosi CM, Bida MN, Bogers JP, Mphahlele MJ. Diversity of HPV types in cancerous and pre-cancerous penile lesions of south African men: implications for future HPV vaccination strategies. J Med Virol. 2014;86(2):257–65.
36. Smith JS, Gilbert PA, Melendy A, Rana RK, Pimenta JM. Age-specific prevalence of human papillomavirus infection in males: a global review. J Adolesc Health. 2011;48(6):540–52.
37. Hakenberg OW, Compérat E, Minhas S, Necchi A, Protzel C, Watkin N et al. EAU – ESTRO – ESUR – SIOG Guidelines on Penile Cancer. *Retrieved from:* https://uroweb.org/guideline/penile-cancer/ accessed 23/09/2021.
38. Flaherty A, Kim T, Giuliano A, Magliocco A, Hakky TS, Pagliaro LC, et al. Implications for human papillomavirus in penile cancer. Urol Oncol. 2014;32(1):53.e1-8.
39. Bezerra AL, Lopes A, Santiago GH, Ribeiro KC, Latorre MR, Villa LL. Human papillomavirus as a prognostic factor in carcinoma of the penis: analysis of 82 patients treated with amputation and bilateral lymphadenectomy. Cancer. 2001;91(12):2315–21.
40. Lont AP, Kroon BK, Horenblas S, Gallee MP, Berkhof J, Meijer CJ, et al. Presence of high-risk human papillomavirus DNA in penile carcinoma predicts favorable outcome in survival. Int J Cancer. 2006;119(5):1078–81.
41. Brown KF, Rumgay H, Dunlop C, Ryan M, Quartly F, Cox A, et al. The fraction of cancer attributable to modifiable risk factors in England, Wales, Scotland, Northern Ireland, and the United Kingdom in 2015. Br J Cancer. 2018;118:1130–41.
42. Hellberg D, Valentin J, Eklund T, Nilsson S. Penile cancer: is there an epidemiological role for smoking and sexual behaviour? Br Med J (Clin Res Ed). 1987;295(6609):1306–8.
43. Tsen HF, Morgenstern H, Mack T, Peters RK. Risk factors for penile cancer: results of a population-based case-control study in Los Angeles County (United States). Cancer Causes Control. 2001;12(3):267–77.
44. Daling JR, Sherman KJ, Hislop TG, Maden C, Mandelson MT, Beckmann AM, Weiss NS. Cigarette smoking and the risk of anogenital cancer. Am J Epidemiol. 1992;135(2):180–9.
45. Harish K, Ravi R. The role of tobacco in penile carcinoma. Br J Urol. 1995;75(3):375–7.

46. Stern RS. PUVA Follow-Up Study. The risk of squamous cell and basal cell cancer associated with psoralen and ultraviolet a therapy: a 30-year prospective study. J Am Acad Dermatol. 2012;66(4):553–62.
47. Stern RS. Genital tumours among men with psoriasis exposed to psoralens and ultraviolet a radiation (PUVA) and ultraviolet B radiation. The photochemotherapy follow-up study. N Engl J Med. 1990;322(16):1093–7.
48. Archier E, Devaux S, Castela E, Gallini A, Aubin F, Le Maître M, et al. Carcinogenic risks of psoralen UV-A therapy and narrowband UV-B therapy in chronic plaque psoriasis: a systematic literature review. J Eur Acad Dermatol Venereol. 2012;26(Suppl 3):22–31.

2 Pathology and Molecular Biology of Penile Cancer

Aiman Haider and Alex Freeman

Learning Objectives

After reading this chapter you will be able to:

- Describe commonly encountered pre cursor penile lesions
- Discuss predisposing lesions related to penile cancer and their histopathological characteristics
- Outline the common histopathological subtypes of penile cancer
- Identify important histopathological features relevant to staging and grading of penile cancer along with their significance in disease outcomes
- List some significant molecular alterations and potential biomarkers used in penile cancer

Introduction

The rarity of penile cancer means that, in non-expert hands, there is a significant risk of misdiagnosis of both the subtype and staging. Accurate staging and grading of tumours are used to determine subsequent clinical management and patient follow up. Different subtypes of penile cancer have been defined, which appear to be associated with variable outcomes leading to treatment strategies [1].

There were significant changes to the 2016 World Health Organization (WHO) classification following the ISUP consultation on Penile Tumours, Boston, in March 2015 [2, 3]. Because of the rarity of penile tumours, this was not a consensus, but an

A. Haider (✉) · A. Freeman
Department of Histopathology, University College London Hospitals NHS Foundation Trust, London, UK
e-mail: aiman.haider@nhs.net

O. Brunckhorst et al. (eds.), *Penile Cancer – A Practical Guide*, Management of Urology, https://doi.org/10.1007/978-3-031-32681-3_2

expert-driven conference aimed at assisting pathologists who do not see these tumours on a regular basis [4]. The fifth edition of the WHO classification of urogenital tumours (WHO "Blue Book"), published in 2022, contains further significant revisions [5].

We attempt to discuss the key updates and pathological features that influence the management and need to be communicated clearly.

Precursor Lesions

Human papillomavirus (HPV)-associated penile intraepithelial neoplasia (PeIN) is a HPV-associated precursor lesion of invasive SCC, whereas differentiated PeIN is an HPV-independent precursor lesion of SCC. The most common HPV-associated PeIN subtypes are the basaloid (undifferentiated, a term that should be avoided) and warty [5] (Table 2.1). From the diagnostic point of view, most penile lesions can be correctly classified using Haematoxylin and eosin (H&E) stain, but immunohistochemical (IHC) or molecular analysis may be helpful in challenging cases.

Patients with HPV-positive tumours have a better prognosis than those with HPV-negative neoplasms, and therefore the identification of the virus in tumour tissue is becoming an important prognostic marker apart from the fact that immunohistochemical (IHC) or molecular analysis may be helpful in challenging cases [6]. The gold-standard test for HPV in tumour tissues is polymerase chain reaction (PCR) but the cost of the technique limits its availability in the majority of laboratories. However, in most cases, p16 has been shown to be an adequate surrogate marker for high-risk HPV [7]. Block-type p16 IHC is the most practical and reliable method to separate HPV associated from HPV-independent penile lesions [5]. Immunohistochemistry for p16 coupled with a proliferation marker Ki-67 is useful in the more challenging cases. Therefore, a panel comprising of p16, p53 and Ki-67 is adequate to correctly diagnose and differentiate benign lesions from pre-malignant lesions.

Immunohistochemistry for p16 is useful to separate differentiated PeIN (Figs. 2.1a–c) which is negative (Fig. 2.2a), whereas the majority of warty, warty-basaloid, and basaloid PeINs (Fig. 2.3a) show diffuse, strong and full thickness (en-bloc) reactivity in the atypical surface squamous epithelium for

Table 2.1 WHO Classification of PeIN

HPV independent	Differentiated
HPV-associated	Basaloid Warty Warty-basaloid
Others	Pleomorphic Spindle Clear cell Pagetoid

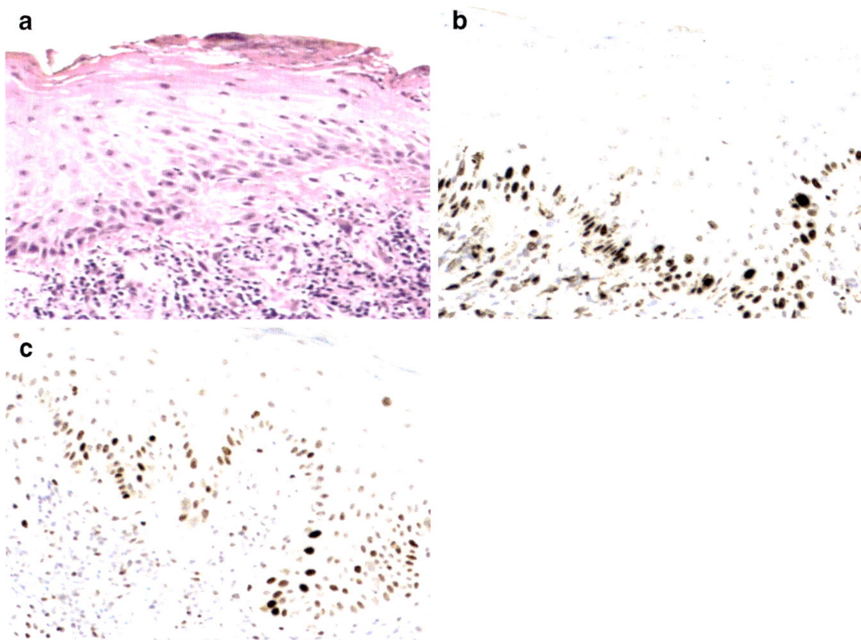

Fig. 2.1 (**a**) Haematoxylin and Eosin stain 20X magnification. Differentiated PeIN with surface maturation and marked atypia of the basal and parabasal keratinocytes. (**b**) MIB-1 stain 20X magnification. Overexpression of proliferation marker in the atypical basal and parabasal cells in differentiated PeIN. (**c**) Immunohistochemistry for p53 (20× magnification) can show 'wild type' staining in differentiated PeIN

p16 [8] (Fig. 2.3b). Differentiated PeIN tends to be associated more commonly with a chronic process such as lichen sclerosus [9]. Recognised different subtypes of differentiated PeIN are hyperplasia like, classic and pleomorphic (Figs. 2.2a–c). Ki-67 is helpful in differentiating the minimal basal atypia of reactive squamous hyperplasia. There is increased basal and parabasal expression with continuous staining in hyperplasia like differentiated PeIN in contrast to the scattered basal cells in benign reactive lesions (Figs. 2.2d and 2.4). Pleomorphic differentiated PeIN can be difficult to differentiate morphologically from undifferentiated PeIN but will be negative on staining for p16 (Fig. 2.2a) [10].

Where available, HPV genotyping can also help contribute to this diagnostic pathway. HPV 16 is the most common genotype and is detected in 71% of basaloid, 56% of warty- basaloid, and 20% of warty PeIN [11].

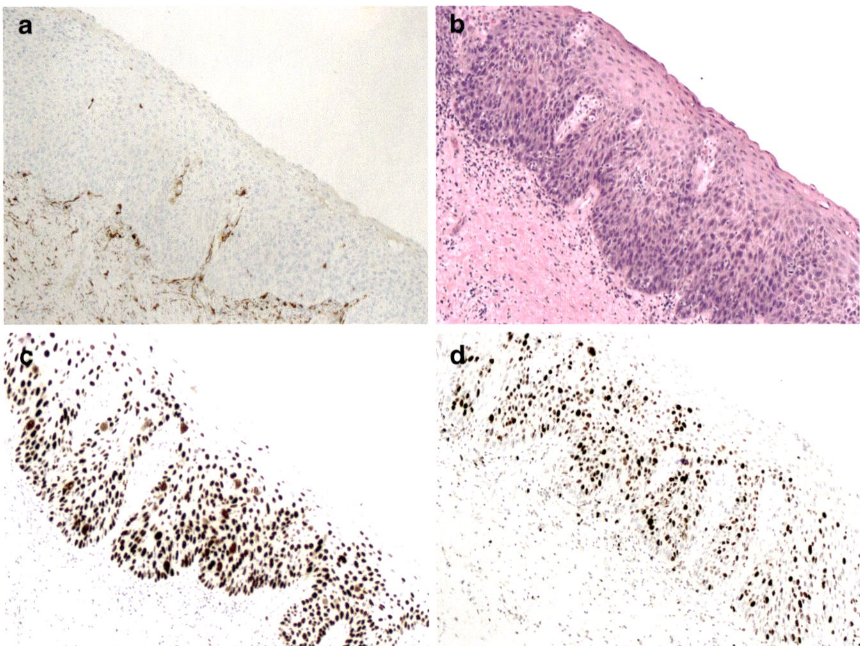

Fig. 2.2 (**a**) Immunohistochemistry for p16. Magnification 20X. No reactivity for p16 in differentiated PeIN. (**b**) Haematoxylin and Eosin stain 10X Magnification. Differentiated PeIN (pleomorphic variant): Marked pleomorphism of the basal and parabasal keratinocytes. There is surface maturation. (**c**) Immunohistochemistry for p53 10X. Differentiated PeIN: Mutant type staining with strong and diffuse overexpression of p53 in basal and parabasal layers. (**d**) Magnification 20X. Immunohistochemistry for MIB-1 overexpression in the atypical basal and parabasal cells of differentiated PeIN

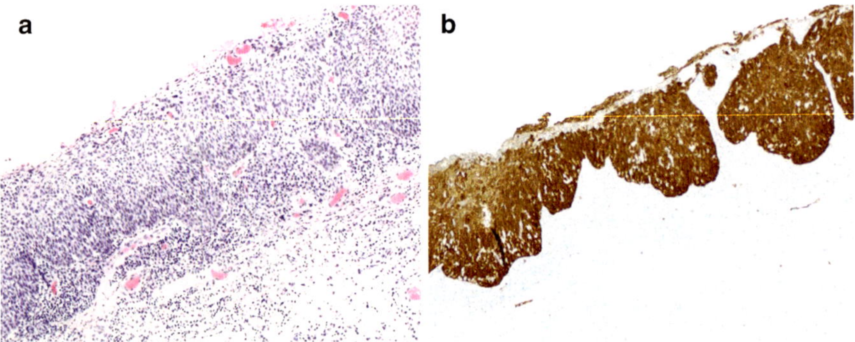

Fig. 2.3 (**a**) Haematoxylin and Eosin stain. Magnification 10X. Undifferentiated PeIN basaloid type. Full thickness atypia of the surface squamous epithelium with a monotonous population of basophilic cells. (**b**) Immunohistochemistry for p16 shows 'en-bloc' strong and diffuse reactivity in undifferentiated PeIN

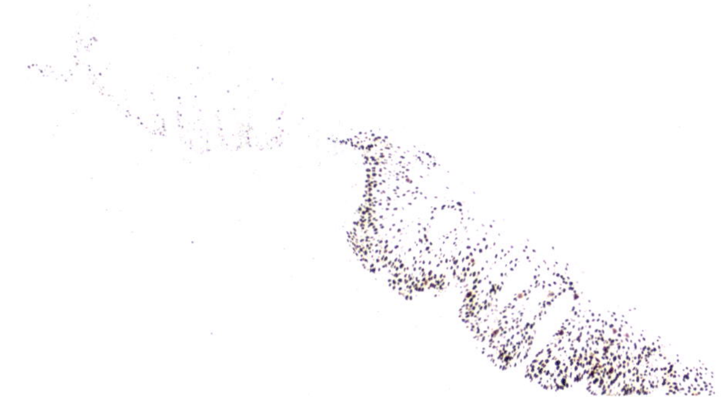

Fig. 2.4 Immunohistochemistry for p53. Magnification 4X. p53 overexpression (diffuse and continuous staining) in differentiated PeIN in contrast to the intermittent basal staining seen in the background surface squamous epithelium

Written reports should indicate the subtype and extent of PeIN and whether or not there is margin involvement.

In difficult cases with cytological abnormalities the category of 'atypia falling short of PeIN' with a recommendation for follow up may be used, to avoid over treatment.

Predisposing Conditions

Condylomata

Condylomata are benign, exophytic, wart-like lesions with koilocytosis and related to infection with low-risk HPV strains, such as HPV 6 and HPV 11 (Figs. 2.5a–c). However, some condylomata show cytologic atypia (Fig. 2.6) and contain high-risk HPV and may be seen in association with PeIN or invasive carcinoma with a variable morphologic spectrum [12]. Penile condyloma types include condyloma acuminatium (typical or atypical) and flat condyloma (typical or atypical).

Immunohistochemistry for p16 is recommended in atypical condylomas to detect the presence of high-risk HPV [13]. However, not all will show staining for p16 and in such cases further in situ hybridization (ISH) or PCR or other molecular techniques may be helpful. Lesions with high-risk HPV should be excised in their entirety and patients need to be more closely followed.

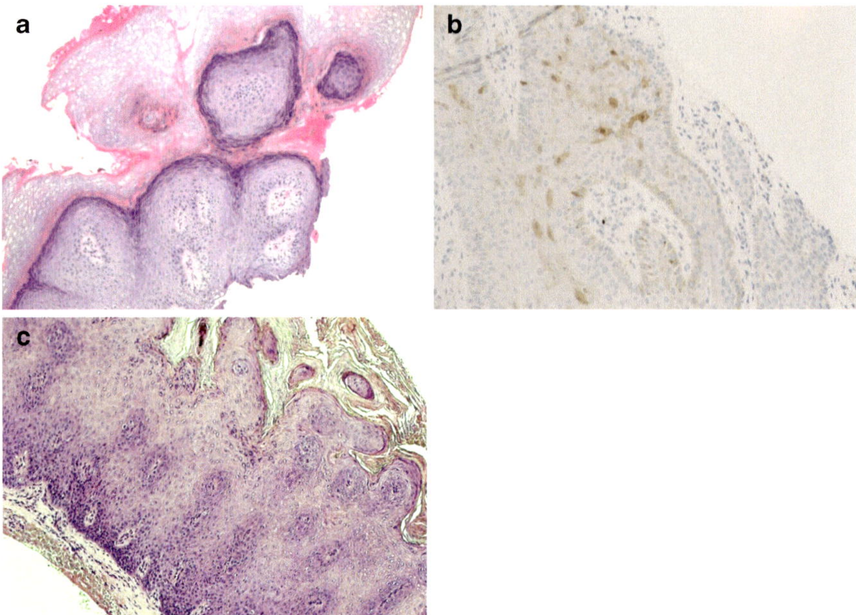

Fig. 2.5 (**a**) Hematocylin and Eosin 10X magnification. Typical Condyloma. Benign squamoproliferative lesion with hyperkeratosis, parakeratosis, acanthosis and papillomatosis of the surface squamous epithelium. (**b**) Immunohistochemistry for p16 shows focal/ scattered reactivity for p16 in the surface keratinocytes. (**c**) Haematoxylin and Eosin 10X. Typical condyloma

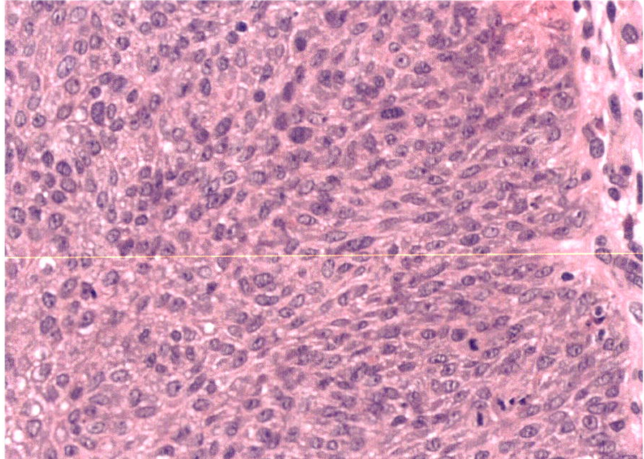

Fig. 2.6 Haemtoxylin and Eosin 40X. Atypical Condyloma. Mild to moderate pleomorphism with frequent mitotic figures

Lichen Sclerosus

The European Association of Urology guidelines identify lichen sclerosus (LSc) as a strong risk factor for penile squamous cell carcinoma but there are also studies to show that it is not associated with increased rates of adverse histopathological features [14, 15]. Differentiated PeINs not linked to HPV, affects elderly men, and is more commonly associated with lichen sclerosus [16, 17]. Histologically, early LSc

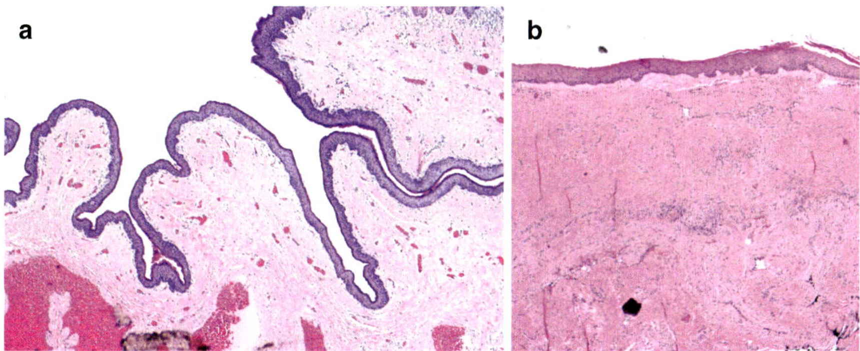

Fig. 2.7 (**a**) Haematoxylin and Eosin 4X. Lichen sclerosus. Attenuation and thinning of the surface squamous epithelium with subepithelial sclerosus and vascular ectasia. (**b**) Haematoxylin and Eosin 4X. Lichen sclerosus. Subepithelial sclerosus and a patchy lichenoid chronic inflammatory cell infiltrate

may show a mild or pronounced band- like CD8 and CD57 positive lymphocytic infiltrate often accompanied by a lymphocytic vasculitis, basal cell vacuolar degeneration and pigment incontinence. As the lesion progresses, subepidermal oedema and sclerosis develops with loss of dermal structures and vascular ectasia (Fig. 2.7a, b) [18]. The histopathology can show varying spectrum of changes depending upon the stage at sampling and it is therefore recommended to examine the specimen in its entirety as focal and early or 'burnt out' changes may be missed.

Penile Cancer

Most malignant tumours of the penis are squamous cell carcinomas (SCCs) originating in the inner mucosal lining of the glans, coronal sulcus, or foreskin. In the 2022 WHO Blue Book, scrotal tumour classification is mentioned separately for the first time [5].

Subtypes

Over 95% of penile cancers are squamous cell carcinomas, with rare instances of sarcomas, melanomas, or neuroendocrine carcinomas (NEC) (including large cell and small cell NEC) [19]. Other malignant lesions of the penis, all much less common than penile SCC, are melanocytic lesions, mesenchymal tumours, lymphomas and metastases. Penile metastases are frequently of prostatic or colorectal origin [14].

Several subtypes have been described and these have different prognostic profiles [20]. Most of these tumours may be diagnosed with H&E histology, but poorly differentiated neoplasms, can be further characterized by immunohistochemical (IHC) and molecular genetic analyses [2]. However, not all positive cases by PCR will be positive by p16 and vice versa, with about a 20% failure in the correlation [3, 21]. Nearly half of penile cancers are human papillomavirus (HPV)-related [22].

The 2016 WHO pathologic classification also adopts categorisation of subtypes of penile SCC as non–HPV-related and HPV-related cases [4, 12, 23]. The 2022 WHO classification followed this paradigm to subclassify tumours into HPV-associated and HPV-independent types (Table 2.2) [24]. It is recommended to report SCC as HPV associated or HPV independent in addition to the histologic diagnosis. If this is not possible, the designation SCC, NOS is acceptable.

A high prevalence of HPV infection is found in basaloid (76%) (Fig. 2.8), mixed warty-basaloid (82%) and warty penile (39%) SCCs while verrucous and papillary penile SCCs are HPV-negative [14].

Subtyping is required as verruciform carcinomas (papillary, warty, or verrucous carcinomas) tend to have better outcomes. Basaloid, acantholytic and sarcomatoid carcinomas are always high grade with a worse prognosis than the usual type of squamous carcinoma and therefore may more readily metastasise to distant sites such as the lung [19]. SCC of the usual type now includes pseudohyperplastic carcinomas and acantholytic/pseudoglandular carcinomas [5]. Verrucous carcinoma is a separate non-metastasising low-grade subtype including carcinoma cuniculatum as a pattern [25].

Up to 30% of tumours may show more than one pattern, all should be recorded in the report. Although not mandatory, reporting a percentage of the poorly differentiated subtypes in such cases is also helpful in guiding management.

Table 2.2 2022 World Health Organization classification of invasive epithelial tumours of the penis and scrotum

HPV associated	Basaloid squamous cell carcinoma Warty carcinoma Clear cell squamous cell carcinoma Lymphoepithelial carcinoma
HPV independent	Squamous cell carcinoma, usual type Verrucous carcinoma (including carcinoma cuniculatum) Papillary squamous cell carcinoma Sarcomatoid squamous cell carcinoma Squamous cell carcinoma, NOS

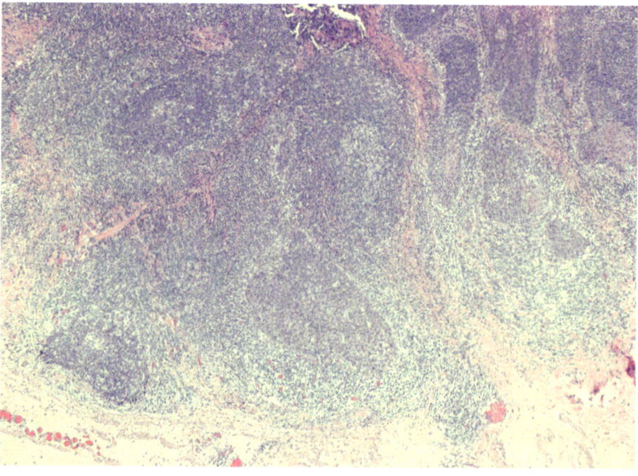

Fig. 2.8 Haematoxylin and Eosin 10X. Basaloid squamous cell carcinoma

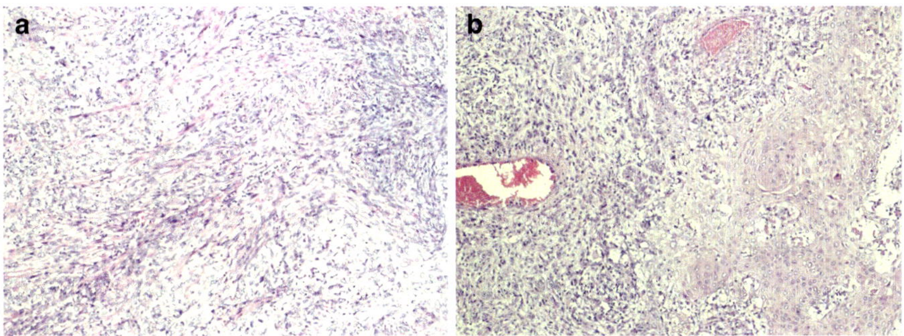

Fig. 2.9 (**a**) Haematoxylin and Eosin stain 10X. Sarcomatoid carcinoma composed of a prominent component of pleomorphic spindle cells in interlacing fascicles. (**b**) Haematoxylin and Eosin stain 10X magnification. An adjacent focus of admixed squamous cell carcinoma helps establish the diagnosis of sarcomatoid carcinoma

Tumour Grading

Differentiation between penile squamous cell carcinoma patients who can benefit from organ-sparing surgery and those at significant risk of lymph node metastasis is based on histopathological prognostic factors including histological grade subtype [26].

The 2016 WHO classification adopted the 3-tier grading method which defines well-, moderately-well and poorly differentiated carcinomas based on the degree of cytological atypia, keratinisation, intercellular bridges, and mitotic activity [4]. Sarcomatoid change is designated as grade 4 and is often in combination with other tumour types (Fig. 2.9a, b). The authors however advise caution in subtyping sarcomatoid variant if seen as focal/isolated cells or in foci adjacent to ulceration. Tumours are graded by the worst area even if this is the minor component.

Although, inconsistencies in concordance can result in under or over treatment of cases, it is important to highlight that recurrent tumours and re-excision specimens for residual tumours from different sites can show different grades.

Tumour Staging

The staging of penile cancer is covered in more detail in in Chap. 4. However, some pertinent issues with regards to pathology are important to consider here. The Royal College of Pathologists recommend the use of The American Joint Committee on Cancer tumour–node–metastasis (AJCC-TNM) staging system eighth edition for penile cancer as it considers factors widely used to predict patient prognoses, guide treatment, and evaluate treatment results. Differences between AJCC and Union Internationale Contre le Cancer eighth Edition

(UICC) staging systems are not minor and using the latter may lead to incorrect reporting of precancerous lesions, superficial tumours, and lymph node staging [27].

In the AJCC eighth edition, Ta disease indicates non-invasive localized squamous cell carcinoma, which allows for inclusion of historical variants other than verrucous carcinoma. This circumvents the confusion caused by UICC in which category pTa was specified as 'non-invasive verrucous carcinoma'. The Royal College of Pathologists guidelines state that this terminology should not be used, as it may falsely lead some pathologists to call verrucous carcinomas of the penis as non-invasive [27].

T1 is subcategorized into T1a and T1b based on the presence of lymphovascular invasion, perineural invasion and high-grade tumour/ poorly differentiated tumour. Urethral invasion is no longer a differentiator between T2 and T3 disease. T2 includes invasion of the corpus spongiosum and T3 involves invasion of the tunica albuginea and corpus cavernosum. The modification of the T2 and T3 stages are reflected in both UICC 8 and AJCC 8. For nodal staging, pN1 has been revised from a single lymph node metastasis to two unilateral inguinal lymph node metastases, while pN2 has been modified to three or more inguinal lymph node metastases [28]. The presence of extra nodal extension indicates an inguinal lymph node stage of pN3, no matter what the extent of the change [27].

Perineurial and Lymphovascular Invasion

Perineurial invasion has been added as an additional prognostic indicator in the AJCC eighth edition [27]. Vascular invasion should be recorded as it is a predictor of nodal metastases [29].

Excision Margins

The presence of microscopic involvement of surgical margins has implications for surgical outcome audit of pre-operative staging and/or surgical technique must be recorded by site and microscopic distance of the tumour from close margins in mm [19]. Providing the actual measurement of lateral extent of individual margins is of value to surgeons in reviewing their techniques. It additionally is part of the required dataset which is recommended to be reported in specimens from penile cancer as per the International Collaboration on Cancer Reporting (ICCR) [30] (Table 2.3).

Table 2.3 ICCR carcinoma of the penis dataset

Recommendation	Element name
Required	• Operative Procedure • Macroscopic Tumour Site • Macroscopic Maximum Tumour Dimensions • Histological Tumour Type • Histological Grade • Microscopic Maximum Tumour Dimensions • Extent of Invasion • Lymphovascular Invasion • Perineural Invasion • Margin Status • Lymph Node Status • Pathological Staging • Primary Tumour T Stage • Regional Lymph Node N Stage
Recommended	• Clinical Information • Tumour Focality • Block Identification Key • Associated Penile Intraepithelial Neoplasia

Table 2.4 Percentage frequency of somatic mutations in penile SCC

Gene	Frequency
TP53	32%
CDKN2A	25%
NOTCH1	17%
PIK3CA	13%
FAT1	25%
CASP8	17%
FBXW7	11%

Molecular Alterations in Penile Cancer

In recent years there has been significant interest in the molecular alterations in penile SCC and several studies have been published highlighting the extent and frequency of these genetic changes. These have been summarised in a recent review paper [31] and the main findings are listed below:

Somatic Mutations

The presence of somatic mutations (Table 2.4) in penile SCC has been extensively examined and involves several genes including tumour suppressor genes (TP53 and CDKN2A), genes involved in cell signalling (NOTCH1, PIK3CA and FAT1) and those involved in apoptosis (CASP8) or acting as cell cycle regulators (FBXW7).

Copy Number Variations

Gains in the MYC gene at 8Q24 have been found in 32% of penile SCC and gains in the EGFR gene at 7p12 have been seen in about 25% of cases. Similar findings have also been reported in head and neck SCC.

Genes Related with HPV Status

Studies have shown a lower mutational load in penile SCC that is HPV-related when compared to cases that are independent of HPV. Furthermore, there appears to be an inverse correlation between HPV positivity and mutations in TP53 and CDKN2A.

Potential Therapeutic Targets

Although many genes have been found to be altered in the pathogenesis of penile SCC, these have been challenging to target separately. Potential therapeutic interventions are typically based on a combination of treatments based on an interaction between a number of signalling pathways. These include:

1. mTOR inhibitors in patients with TP53 mutation and stimulated PI3K signalling pathway.
2. PARP inhibitors in patients with defective DNA repair pathways.
3. Combination of PI3K and mTOR inhibitors in NOTCH1 mutated tumours.

Markers of Penile Cancer Progression and Metastasis

The genetic alterations seen in penile SCC may be involved either in primary carcinogenesis, tumour progression or metastatic spread [32]:

1. Primary carcinogenesis
   A. Genes upregulated by inflammation – COX2, PGE2
   B. Tumour suppressor genes – p53, p16, PTEN
   C. Oncogenes – HPV E6 / 7, MYC
   D. Apoptosis – bcl2, p53, telomerases
2. Proliferation and invasion
   A. Growth factors / receptors- EGFR, Her3, VEGF, PI3K, PTEN, AKT
   B. Epithelial / mesenchymal - MMP2 / MMP9, E cadherin, Glut1
   C. Cell cycle – Ki67
3. Metastasis
   A. Metastasis suppressor genes – KAI1, Nm23H1

The identification of the stage of tumorigenesis in which these particular genes are involved may result in new small molecular target agents that may stop the local growth or spread of penile SCC and allow the prospect of curative treatment in affected patients.

Summary

In conclusion, surgeons need to be aware of the updated changes in the classification of penile tumours, the significance and nomenclature of PeIN, the pathological risk factors and the differences highlighted in the updated AJCC and UICC stagings. Patients with penile cancer should be referred to a specialist centre, with any diagnostic slides and/or blocks made available for expert review prior to subsequent treatment planning by the specialist team to ensure correct diagnosis, subtyping, grading, and staging. Standardized structured reporting guidelines and discussion at the supra-regional multidisciplinary team meetings lead to optimal management decisions taken and subsequently better oncological outcomes and patient survival. Communication with high quality reports and understanding of clinicians of what constitutes an adequate report, is the key to ensure proper management of these patients.

Key Points

- Due to its rarity, it is important to have specialist pathological expertise available to evaluate histopathological, immunohistochemical and molecular genetic features of penile specimens.
- Important pathological features to consider include presence of precursor lesions and predisposing lesions such as lichen sclerosus and condylomatous changes.
- Knowledge of subtyping of both HPV and non-HPV related penile cancers is important due to their differing prognostic profiles.
- Other important prognostic features on pathology include grade, stage, presence of perineurial, lymphovascular invasion and excision margins.
- Various potential biomarkers exist including Ki67, SCC antigen e cadherin and p53.

Revisions Questions

Multiple Choice Questions

1. What is the causative agent for condyloma acuminatum?
   (a) HSV
   (b) HPV 6 and 11
   (c) E. coli
   (d) Schistosoma

2. Which of the following are HPV related pre-cancerous conditions (Choose all that apply)?
   (a) Warty undifferentiated PeIN.
   (b) Basaloid undifferentiated PeIN
   (c) Differentiated PeIN
   (d) Paget's disease
3. Which immunohistochemical marker is a surrogate for HPV in the tissue
   (a) P53
   (b) P63
   (c) P16
   (d) KI-67
4. Which of the following is recommended for pathological staging of penile squamous cell carcinoma and considers pathological risk factors for appropriate management decisions?
   (a) AJCC 8th edition
   (b) AJCC 7th edition
   (c) UICC 8th edition
   (d) All of the above
   (e) None of the above

Viva Cases

Case 1

A 51-year-old man presents with a flat white lesion with irregular and indistinct borders on the glans. Histopathology shows hyperkeratosis, parakeratosis, and prominent cytological atypia in the basal keratinocytes. The background skin shows features in keeping with lichen sclerosus. The atypia extends to the peripheral limit.

A. What are the differential diagnoses and key points indicated in the history and pathology?

Case 2

Following a previous diagnosis of squamous cell carcinoma which was treated by glans resurfacing, a 75-year-old man presents with a recurrent ulcerated fungating tumour of the neo-glans involving the coronal sulcus. Sectioning of the specimen received in pathology shows deep invasion of the cavernosum. Histopathology shows a poorly differentiated grade 3–4 squamous cell carcinoma composed predominantly of spindle cells with increased atypical mitosis, necrosis, multinucleated cells, and multiple foci of perineurial and lymphovascular invasion.

A. What is the subtype of cancer in discussion and the key points related to this subtype?

Answers

Multiple Choice Questions

1. **B.** Condyloma acuminatum in the majority of cases is caused by low risk HPV genotypes 6 and 11
2. **A and B.** Undifferentiated PeIN has been very strongly related to oncogenic HPV infection resulting from the integration of viral genome into the DNA of the host cell, leading to oncogene overexpression and cell proliferation. This is morphologicaly of three types; warty, basaloid and warty-basaloid.
3. **C.** Strong and diffuse nuclear expression of p16 is a strong predictor for the presence of HPV (high risk) in penile neoplasia.
4. **A.** Except for the modification of the T2 and T3 stages, which are the same in UICC 8 and AJCC 8, the advances documented in the literature do not seem to have been considered in UICC 8.

Viva Cases

Case 1

A. Important Discussion Points to cover:
   - Type of pre-cancerous and predisposing lesions
   - Differentiated versus undifferentiated PeIN (HPV related)
   - Association of lichen sclerosus and differentiated PeIN
   - The value of p16 (negative in differentiated PeIN) and Ki-67 (overexpression in the basal and parabasal layers) in the diagnosis of pre-cancerous lesions
   - Follow up and close surveillance advised in cases of margin involvement. Asses for presence of multifocal lesions.
   - Concomitant penile carcinoma if present, is usually low grade of ususal, verrucous, papillary and pseudohyperplastic type.

Case 2

A. Important discussion points to cover include:
   - Sarcomatoid carcinoma is a rare and aggressive variant of squamous cell carcinoma.
   - Presence of adjacent squamous cell carcinoma or PeIN helps establish a diagnosis.
   - Spindle cell should comprise 30% of the tumour to qualify for the diagnosis.
   - Any history of previous treatment (radiotherapy) should be documented.
   - This tumour is pT3 and shows perineurial and lymphovascular invasion which are all adverse pathological risk factors.
   - These cases have a high mortality rate with increased risk of haematogenous and lymph node metastases as well as local recurrence.

Test your learning and check your understanding of this book's contents: use the "Springer Nature Flashcards" app to access questions using ▶ https://sn.pub/1r7Om8. To use the app, please follow the instructions in chapter 1.

References

1. Epstein JI, Cubilla AL, Humphrey PA. Tumours of the prostate gland, seminal vesicles, penis and scrotum. Washington, DC: Armed Forces Institute of Pathology; 2011. p. 405–611.
2. Canete-Portillo S, Velazquez EF, Kristiansen G, Egevad L, Grignon D, Chaux A, Cubilla AL. Report From the International Society of Urological Pathology (ISUP) consultation conference on molecular pathology of urogenital cancers V. Am J Surg Pathol. 2020;44(7):e80–6. https://doi.org/10.1097/PAS.0000000000001477.
3. Cañete-Portillo S, Sanchez D, Alemany L, et al. The relative value of P16 for HPV detection in penile carcinomas. A study of 219 of the most common HPV-related neoplasms. Mod Pathol. 2019;32:24–5.
4. Cubilla AL, Velazquez EF, Amin MB, Epstein J, Berney DM, Corbishley CM, Members of the ISUP Penile Tumor Panel. The World Health Organisation 2016 classification of penile carcinomas: a review and update from the International Society of Urological Pathology expert-driven recommendations. Histopathology. 2018;72(6):893–904. https://doi.org/10.1111/his.13429. Epub 2018 Feb 9
5. Moch H, Amin MB, Berney DM, Comperat EM, Gill AJ, Hartmann A, Menon S, Raspollini MR, Rubin MA, Srigley JR, Hoon Tan P, Tickoo SK, Tsuzuki T, Turajlic S, Cree I, Netto GJ. The 2022 World Health Organization classification of tumours of the urinary system and male genital organs-part a: renal, penile, and testicular tumours. Eur Urol. 2022;S0302-2838(22):02467-8. https://doi.org/10.1016/j.eururo.2022.06.016. Epub ahead of print
6. Djajadiningrat RS, Jordanova ES, Kroon BK, et al. Human papillomavirus prevalence in invasive penile cancer and association with clinical outcome. J Urol. 2015;193:526–31.
7. Cubilla AL, Lloveras B, Alejo M, et al. Value of p16(INK)^4(a) in the pathology of invasive penile squamous cell carcinomas: a report of 202 cases. Am J Surg Pathol. 2011;35:253–61.
8. Chaux A, Velazquez EF, Amin A, et al. Distribution and characterization of subtypes of penile intraepithelial neoplasia and their association with invasive carcinomas: a pathological study of 139 lesions in 121 patients. Hum Pathol. 2012;43:1020–7.
9. Soskin A, Vieillefond A, Carlotti A, Plantier F, Chaux A, Ayala G, Velazquez EF, Cubilla AL. Warty/basaloid penile intraepithelial neoplasia is more prevalent than differentiated penile intraepithelial neoplasia in nonendemic regions for penile cancer when compared with endemic areas: a comparative study between pathologic series from Paris and Paraguay. Hum Pathol. 2012;43(2):190–6. https://doi.org/10.1016/j.humpath.2011.04.014. Epub 2011 Aug 10
10. Cañete-Portillo S, Sanchez D, Cabanas ML, et al. The value and limitations of P16 and Ki67 immunostains in the diagnosis and subtyping of differentiated penile intraepithelial neoplasia (DPeIN). Mod Pathol. 2020;33:886–7.
11. Fernández-Nestosa MJ, Guimerà N, Sanchez DF, et al. Human papillomavirus (HPV) genotypes in condylomas, intraepithelial neoplasia, and invasive carcinoma of the penis using laser capture microdissection (LCM)-PCR: a study of 191 lesions in 43 patients. Am J Surg Pathol. 2017;41:820–32.
12. Cubilla AL. Tumors of the penis. In: Epstein JI, Cubilla AL, Magi- Galluzzi C, editors. Tumors of the prostate gland, seminal vesicles, penis, and scrotum. 5th ed. Wahsington DC: American Registry of Pathology/Armed Forces Institute of Pathology; 2020.

13. Sudenga SL, Ingles DJ, Pierce Campbell CM, et al. Genital human papillomavirus infection progression to external genital lesions: the HIM study. Eur Urol. 2016;69:166–73.
14. Hakenberg OW, Compérat EM, Minhas S, Necchi A, Protzel C, Watkin N. EAU guidelines on penile cancer: 2014 update. Eur Urol. 2015;67(1):142–50. https://doi.org/10.1016/j.eururo.2014.10.017. Epub 2014 Nov 1
15. Philippou P, Shabbir M, Ralph DJ, Malone P, Nigam R, Freeman A, Muneer A, Minhas S. Genital lichen sclerosus/balanitis xerotica obliterans in men with penile carcinoma: a critical analysis. BJU Int. 2013;111(6):970–6. https://doi.org/10.1111/j.1464-410X.2012.11773.x. Epub 2013 Jan 29
16. Moguelet P, Compérat EM. Les néoplasies intraépithéliales peniennes [penile intraepithelial neoplasia]. Ann Pathol. 2022;42(1):15–9. https://doi.org/10.1016/j.annpat.2021.04.005. French. Epub 2021 Dec 2
17. Cañete-Portillo S, Sanchez DF, Fernández-Nestosa MJ, Piris A, Zarza P, Oneto S, Gonzalez Stark L, Lezcano C, Ayala G, Rodriguez I, Hoang MP, Mihm MC, Cubilla AL. Continuous spatial sequences of lichen Sclerosus, penile intraepithelial neoplasia, and invasive carcinomas: a study of 109 cases. Int J Surg Pathol. 2019;27(5):477–82. https://doi.org/10.1177/1066896918820960. Epub 2019 Jan 7
18. Sewell A, Oxley J. An overview of benign and premalignant lesions of the foreskin. Diagn Histopathol. 2019;25(10):390–7.ISSN 1756-2317. https://doi.org/10.1016/j.mpdhp.2019.07.002.
19. Corbishley C, Oxley J, Shanks J, Brenden T. The Royal College of Pathologists. Dataset for penile and distal urethral cancer histopathology reports. July 2015.
20. Thomas A, Necchi A, Muneer A, Tobias-Machado M, Tran ATH, Van Rompuy AS, Spiess PE, Albersen M. Penile cancer. Nat Rev Dis Primers. 2021;7(1):11. https://doi.org/10.1038/s41572-021-00246-5.
21. Olesen TB, Sand FL, Rasmussen CL, Albieri V, Toft BG, Norrild B, Munk C, Kjær SK. Prevalence of human papillomavirus DNA and p16^{INK4a} in penile cancer and penile intraepithelial neoplasia: a systematic review and meta-analysis. Lancet Oncol. 2019;20(1):145–58. https://doi.org/10.1016/S1470-2045(18)30682-X. Epub 2018 Dec 17
22. Alemany L, Cubilla A, Halec G, et al. Role of human papillomavirus in penile carcinomas worldwide. Eur Urol. 2016;69:953–61.
23. Moch H, Humphrey PA, Ulbright TM, Reuter VE. WHO classification of tumours of the urinary system and male genital organs. 4th ed. Lyon: IARC Press; 2015.
24. WHO. Classification of tumours of the urinary system and male genital organs. 5th ed. Lyon, France: International Agency for Research on Cancer; 2022.
25. Barreto JE, Velazquez EF, Ayala E, Torres J, Cubilla AL. Carcinoma Cuniculatum: a distinctive variant of penile squamous cell carcinoma: report of 7 cases. Am J Surg Pathol. 2007;31(1):71–5. https://doi.org/10.1097/01.pas.0000213401.72569.22.
26. Dorofte L, Grélaud D, Fiorentino M, Giunchi F, Ricci C, Franceschini T, Riefolo M, Davidsson S, Carlsson J, Lillsunde Larsson G, Karlsson MG. Low level of interobserver concordance in assessing histological subtype and tumor grade in patients with penile cancer may impair patient care. Virchows Arch. 2022;480(4):879–86. https://doi.org/10.1007/s00428-021-03249-5. Epub 2021 Dec 10
27. Delahunt B, Egevad L, Samaratunga H, Varma M, Verrill C, Cheville J, Kristiansen G, Corbishley C, Berney DM. UICC drops the ball in the 8th edition TNM staging of urological cancers. Histopathology. 2017;71(1):5–11. https://doi.org/10.1111/his.13200.
28. Khalil MI, Kamel MH, Dhillon J, Master V, Davis R, Hajiran AJ, Spiess PE. What you need to know: updates in penile cancer staging. World J Urol. 2021;39(5):1413–9. https://doi.org/10.1007/s00345-020-03302-z. Epub 2020 Jun 22
29. Slaton JW, Morgenstern N, Levy DA, Santos MW Jr, Tamboli P, Ro JY, et al. Tumor stage, vascular invasion and the percentage of poorly differentiated cancer: independent prognosticators for inguinal lymph node metastasis in penile squamous cancer. J Urol. 2001;165:1138–42.

30. Corbishley C, Chaux A, Colecchia M, Cubilla AL, Shanks J, Velazquez EF, Watkin N, Srigley JR. Carcinoma of the penis and distal urethra histopathology reporting guide. 1st ed. Sydney, Australia: International Collaboration on Cancer Reporting; 2017. ISBN: 978-1-925687-05-7
31. Ribera-Cortada I, Guerrero-Pineda J, Trias I, Veloza L, Garcia A, Marimon L, Diaz-Mercedes S, Alamo JR, Rodrigo-Calvo MT, Vega N, Lopez del Campo R, Parra-Medina R, Ajami T, Martinez A, Reig O, Ribal Maria J, Corral-Molina JM, Jares P, Ordi J, Rakislova N. Pathogenesis of penile squamous cell carcinoma: molecular update and systematic review. Int J Mol Sci. 2022;23:251.
32. Protzel C, Spiess PE. Molecular research in penile cancer—lessons learned from the past and bright horizons of the future? Int J Mol Sci. 2013;14:19494–505.

Imaging Techniques Used in Penile Cancer

3

Alex Kirkham and Adam Retter

Learning Objectives

After reading this chapter you will be able to:

- Describe the commonly used imaging modalities for the local staging of penile cancer disease
- Outline imaging options for the nodal staging of disease
- Define methods for evaluating presence of metastatic disease in patients
- Review relevant anatomy on imaging modalities utilised to stage patients
- Apply common current guidelines for the imaging of patients with suspected and confirmed penile cancer

A. Kirkham (✉) · A. Retter
Department of Radiology, University College London Hospitals NHS Foundation Trust, London, UK

O. Brunckhorst et al. (eds.), *Penile Cancer – A Practical Guide*, Management of Urology, https://doi.org/10.1007/978-3-031-32681-3_3

Introduction

Imaging can be used to provide information on each component of the TNM staging of penile cancer and may therefore be useful for surgical planning and estimating prognosis. Recommendations for the use of imaging are included in the most recent (2018) EAU guidelines on the management of penile cancer [1], and we aim to describe the (a) radiological anatomy and (b) the technical aspects and performance characteristics of the most commonly used techniques. We will begin by describing the techniques for imaging the penis itself, and then move on to nodal and metastatic disease detection and protocols for surveillance after treatment.

Imaging the Penis: Local Staging, Clinical Examination, Ultrasound, and MRI

The first important point is that the penis is a superficial organ, with (a) the great majority of tumours occurring in the distal part and (b) skip lesions being rare and usually occurring with advanced disease. Therefore, in the great majority of cases clinical assessment is accurate in estimating the size and location of the tumour: it does not follow inevitably that any imaging technique will be superior, or cost-effective. It is not enough to show that MRI can be moderately accurate in staging the local disease [2]: rather, the technique must be more accurate than palpation *and* improve our treatment. With this in mind, we will briefly describe the anatomy of the penis relevant to imaging, and the technique for ultrasound and MRI. CT is useful in nodal staging (where there is usually adequate contrast between soft tissue nodes and surrounding fat) but its soft tissue contrast is too poor to be used routinely for the penis itself.

The Anatomy of the Penis as Seen on MRI

T2 images are the mainstay of MRI imaging in most parts of the body, as they usually show the best contrast between different soft tissues. In the penis the contrast between the high signal contents of the glans, corpus spongiosum and corpora cavernosa and the lower signal fascial layers is much better seen on T2 than T1 sequences [3].

The corpora cavernosa and the corpus spongiosum are surrounded by a T2 low signal fibrous sheath, the tunica albuginea (Fig. 3.1). Although this has inner (circular) and outer (longitudinal) layers, they are not distinguishable on imaging. Buck's fascia lies just outside and although it may be separable surgically, in most cases it appears as part of the T2 low signal tunical layer [4] (Fig. 3.2). In the dorsal midline the deep dorsal vessels lie deep to Buck's fascia, and it may be possible to distinguish them here, with some higher signal connective tissue, but in practice even this anatomy is often hard to see. The normal T2 low signal tunica/Buck's

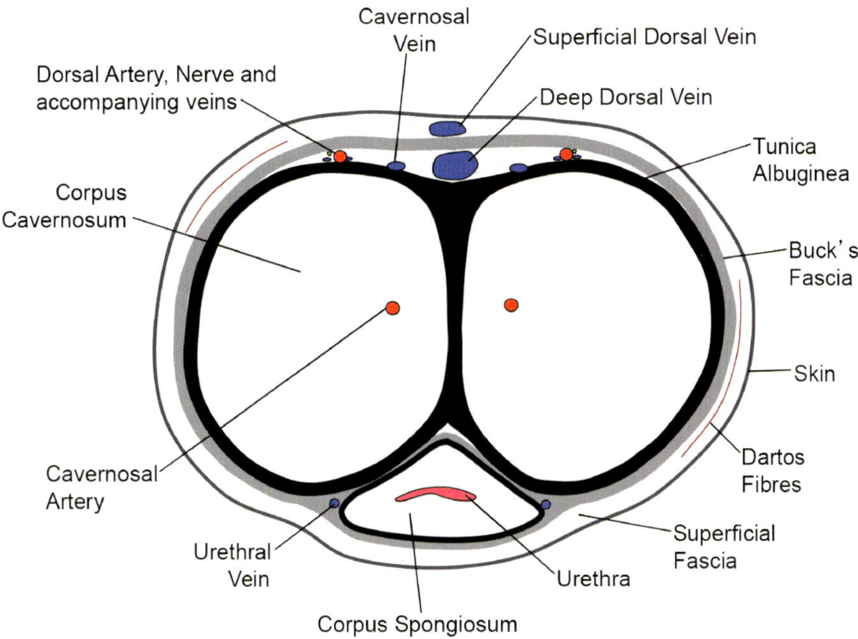

Fig. 3.1 Penile anatomy visible on MRI and ultrasound. Axial section at mid shaft. With permission from Muneer A and Horenblas S, *Textbook of Penile Cancer*, Springer International Publishing

layer is always thicker over the corpora cavernosa than spongiosum. In the glans it is hard to define, fusing completely with the subepithelial connective tissue toward the tip.

Outside Buck's fascia are the superficial vessels in a looser connective tissue layer, sometimes called the Dartos fascia, continuous with Colle's fascia of the perineum and continuing thin dartos muscle fibres. Haematoma deep to Buck's fascia is confined to the penis, but if in the superficial fascial layer can extend to scrotum and abdominal wall. The bulb is covered by a T2 low signal bulbocavernosus muscle layer, and the crura as they lie against the ischium are covered medially by the ischiocavernosus muscle.

The cavernosal arteries are usually seen as *signal voids* on T2 sequences. On enhanced images they are usually of high signal, and the surrounding contrast radiates axially outwards, and from proximal to distal (with different patterns sometimes seen in infarction, tumour and metastasis). The urethra is usually seen as a flattened intermediate T2 signal structure within the corpus spongiosum, but can be hard to identify reliably, especially in the context of tumour [5].

On T1 weighted images, enhancing tissues are of high signal. In any study with contrast (and especially in the case of trauma or tumour) it is important to obtain pre-contrast images because blood products are often also high in T1 signal and can mimic enhancement. Diffusion-weighted imaging has been useful in the prostate and has recently been applied to penile cancer, but because it has not yet been shown to be clinically useful, we will not describe it in detail [6].

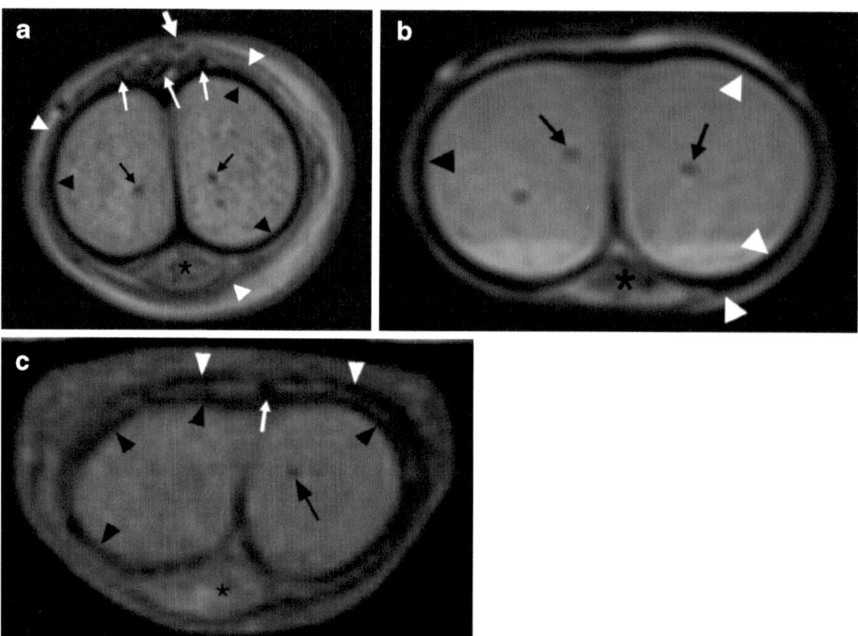

Fig. 3.2 Axial T2-weighted (**a**, **b**) and T1-weighted (**c**) images through the penis in different patients after intracavernosal alprostadil. Note the differing conspicuity of Buck's fascia and the dorsal vessels: clearly visible in patients (**a**, **c**) but not (**b**). *Black arrowheads* mark the tunica albuginea, and *white arrowheads* Buck's fascia. The *thick white arrow* shows the superficial dorsal vein in (**a**), and the thinner *white arrows* the deep dorsal vessels. The cavernosal arteries are marked by *black arrows*. The urethra, lying in the middle of the corpus spongiosum, is marked by an *asterisk*. Note the layering of signal within the corpora cavernosa in (**b**), a normal finding. With permission from Muneer A and Horenblas S, *Textbook of Penile Cancer*, Springer International Publishing

Anatomy on Ultrasound

As in the scrotum, the dependent part of the penis (and in most cases all of the crura and bulb) can be imaged with a high frequency (10 MHz or greater) probe, giving a spatial resolution (usually under 0.3 mm) that easily exceeds MRI or CT. As on MRI, the tunica albuginea and Buck's fascia appear as one layer, this time echogenic and 'bright' (Figs. 3.3 and 3.4). If the penis is rotated, it can be difficult to distinguish the corpus spongiosum and corpora cavernosa, which have contents of similar echogenicity. However, the urethra is usually visible in the former. In the glans the subepithelial connective tissue and tunica albuginea become indistinguishable, making the distinction between T1 and T2 tumours challenging. Cavernosal vessels are easily seen.

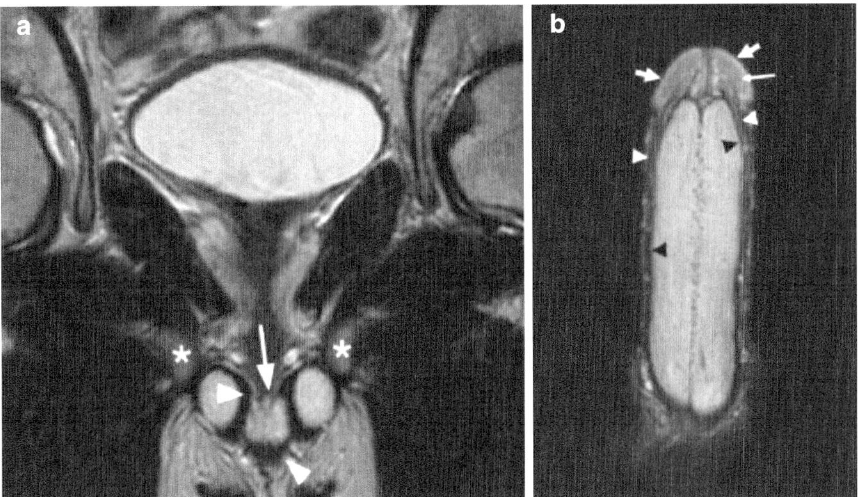

Fig. 3.3 T2-weighted coronal section through the base (**a**) and shaft (**b**) of the penis after intracavernosal alprostadil. In (**a**) a *white arrowhead* marks the ischiocavernosus muscle, and a *black arrowhead* the bulbocavernosus. A *white arrow* shows the urethra entering the bulb. Inferior pubic rami are marked by *asterisks*. In (**b**), a *black arrowhead* marks the tunica albuginea and a *white arrowhead* Buck's fascia. The glans is well seen (*thick white arrows*). With permission from Muneer A and Horenblas S, *Textbook of Penile Cancer*, Springer International Publishing

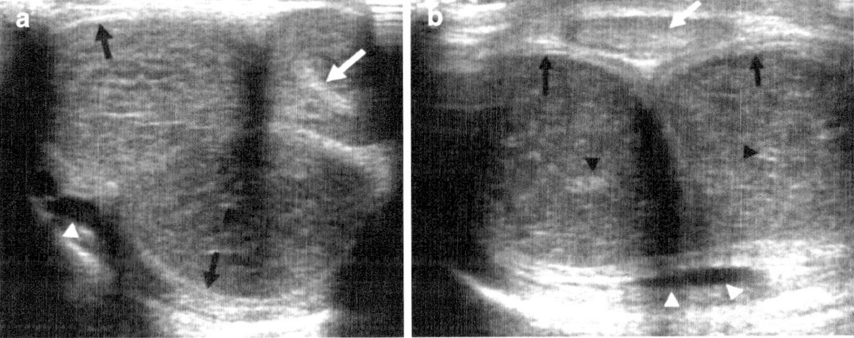

Fig. 3.4 Two axial images of the shaft of the tumescent penis: the first (**a**) taken at an angle of 45° to avoid diffraction artifact, and the second (**b**), in the standard transverse plane with the probe ventral. The urethra (*white arrow*) is sometimes seen well within the corpus spongiosum. Tunica albuginea and Buck's fascia (*black arrows*) appear as one echogenic layer, thickest around the corpora cavernosa. *White arrowheads* show superficial vessels, and *black arrowheads* the cavernosal vessels. With permission from Muneer A and Horenblas S, *Textbook of Penile Cancer*, Springer International Publishing

Table 3.1 Additional sequences used in MRI

Sequence	Utility
T2 images in 3 planes	Mainstay of imaging and always used
T1 imaging	(a) Baseline sequence before giving contrast (b) Useful for defining marrow fat in possible bony involvement
STIR imaging or T2 fat saturated images	(a) To detect oedema, often in the case of infection / abscess (b) To screen for bony metastases
Enhanced T1 images	(a) *Sometimes* (but not routinely) useful to define tumour and metastases. (b) To define vascular anatomy (although often well seen on T2) (c) To detect infarction (rarely indicated in the context of penile cancer)
Diffusion weighted imaging	Under investigation Not used routinely

Imaging Techniques: MRI

The penis is positioned in the anatomical position, against the abdominal wall (though others position dependently to reduce breathing artefact) [7]. This enables accurate measurement of length [8] and the best opportunity to define the relationship of the tumour to other structures. The mainstay of MRI imaging is T2 sequences, and for many scans *these are all that are required.* We use a field of view of 20–24 cm, slices of 3 mm and an in plane resolution between 0.7 and 1 mm. Additional sequences can be added for different indications (Table 3.1), but we do not routinely use contrast enhancement (which lengthens scan times and requires cannulation) as it has not been shown to improve accuracy [9].

Ultrasound, and the Need for Tumescence

Ultrasound has a higher theoretical resolution with MRI but is (a) more operator-dependent, (b) produces images which are harder to interpret by non-radiologists and (c) has less intrinsic contrast between tumour and the normal anatomical structures of the penis (although this is variable). However, performed by someone with an interest in the field and especially with the use of artificial erection (as discussed below) it can produce excellent images: we would assert that a specialist penile cancer service could operate perfectly well with routine use of ultrasound, reserving MRI for occasional challenging cases.

One area of controversy is the use of agents to produce artificial erection. Tumescence distends the corpora cavernosa, with several benefits: (a) producing a thin and usually smooth appearance to the tunical / Buck's layer, (b) making the contents of the corpora uniformly high in signal on MRI, increasing contrast with tumour and (c) makes positioning in the true anatomical plane easier (Fig. 3.5). We (and others) [5] find these benefits compelling, though others do not [8]. We do not produce erection for very large tumours, where it might be uncomfortable and is

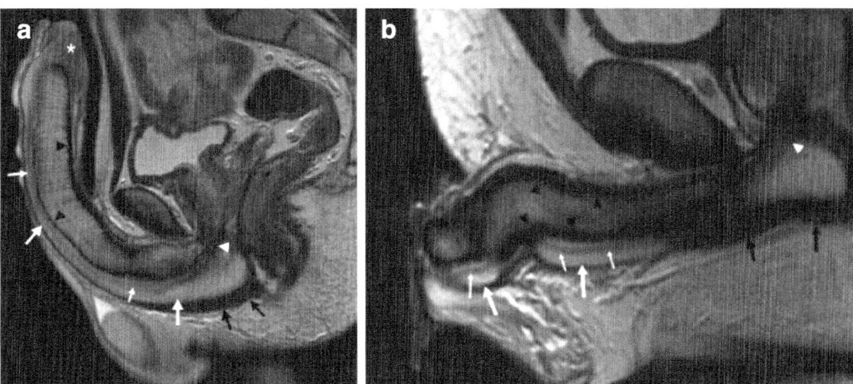

Fig. 3.5 T2-weighted sagittal section close to the midline (**a**) after intracavernosal alprostadil and (**b**) without tumescence. *Black arrows* mark the tunica albuginea, large *white arrows* the corpus spongiosum, small *white arrows* the urethra within it, and *black arrows* the bulbocavernosus muscle. The *white arrow head* marks the entry of the urethra into the roof of the bulb. An *asterisk* marks the glans. The 'corrugated' appearance of the corpus cavernosum in (**a**) is because of the midline intercavernosal septum. Note the considerably thicker tunica albuginea in the detumescent state, and the lower signal in the corpus cavernosum; the glans is not in the midline sagittal plane. With permission from Muneer A and Horenblas S, *Textbook of Penile Cancer*, Springer International Publishing

unlikely to significantly improve accuracy. The normal dose is 5–10 mcg of Caverject (depending on age and erectile function). The risk of priapism is small (1% in erectile dysfunction of mixed cause [10] and not occurring at all in a recent series of 100 patients with penile cancer [5]). If it does occur, aspiration is often effective and can be supplemented by intracavernosal injection of phenylephrine [11].

MRI and Ultrasound for Primary Staging

The great majority of penile cancers are squamous cell carcinomas (SCC), although melanoma, sarcomas and lymphoma have been reported [7]. Metastases are rare and varied in origin, though most likely to occur from a bladder primary [12]. On MRI, tumour is usually intermediate in signal: higher than the low signal fascial layers but (especially in the case of artificial erection) lower than the high signal contents of the corpora cavernosa (Figs. 3.5 and 3.6). On ultrasound the fascial layers are bright, and tumour is usually relatively hypoechoic, though sometimes heterogenous.

Local staging has potential implications for surgical planning and prognosis. However, (a) definitive staging is obtained with the surgical histology and provides the most accurate prognostic information and (b) although decisions about the surgical approach may be informed by the imaging, no technique has been shown to be fully accurate. Given that the mainstay treatment is surgical, decisions about the extent of the resection will also be made with the operative findings (and potentially,

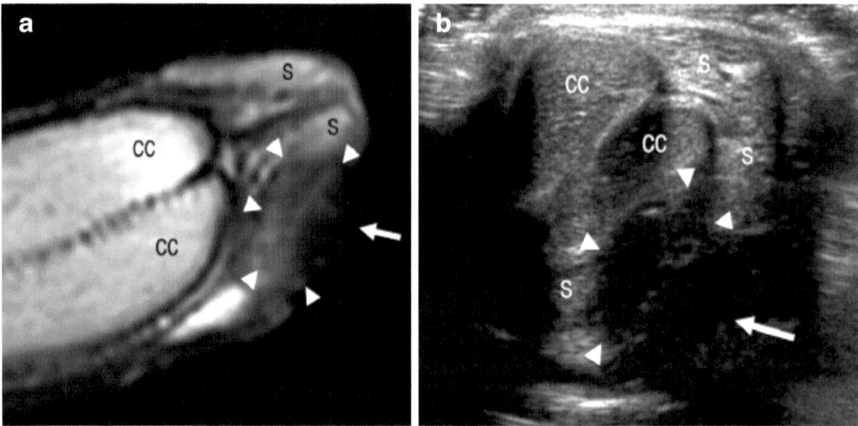

Fig. 3.6 Ulcerating lesion on the glans (*white arrowheads*, with a *white arrow* showing the ulcerated part), pT2 on histology and correctly called T2 on MRI (**a**) and ultrasound (**b**). CC marks corpus cavernosum, and S the spongiosal part of the glans. Note that on MR the underlying high signal of the spongiosal tissue of the glans is altered by the tumour, although the tips of the cavernosa are well seen and not involved. The ultrasound confirms involvement of the spongiosal tissue of the glans but not the corpora cavernosa. With permission from Muneer A and Horenblas S, Textbook of Penile Cancer, Springer International Publishing

frozen section histology [13]). Imaging, therefore, may be useful for counselling the patient but will not necessarily indicate the definitive surgical approach.

Whilst most previous studies used pre-2018 TNM definitions, they provide a good estimate of accuracy of MRI with artificial erection. The largest of these from 2015 found the sensitivity and specificity for invasion of the tunica albuginea to be 82% and 79%, and for urethral involvement, 63% and 87% [5]. However, more recent evidence from 54 patients without caverject showed sensitivity and specificity of 96% and 94% for spongiosal involvement, and 88% and 98% for cavernosal involvement with urethral involvement sometimes overestimated (a positive predictive value of 63%) [8]. In a study using a consensus of radiologist opinion and IV contrast, these are good results, raising the possibility that intracavernosal agents may not be necessary in routine practice.

Perhaps the most valuable study of both ultrasound and MRI, published in 2016, compares 200 patients, with intracavernosal agents and correlation with operative histology [14]. MRI had sensitivity and specificity of 74% and 98.5%, and ultrasound 97% and 96% for cavernosal involvement. This reinforces our impression that if ultrasound is available, MRI is not essential for the adequate management of penile cancer (as discussed in sections below, CT can be used for nodal and metastatic disease detection). Lastly, when comparing physical examination, MRI and ultrasound a previous study actually found physical examination to be the most accurate estimator of the size of the tumour and detected most cases of cavernosal invasion with no false positives [15]. Whilst not investigated in larger studies of ultrasound and MRI, this study although old raises an important question about the necessity of routine imaging for local staging (Fig. 3.7).

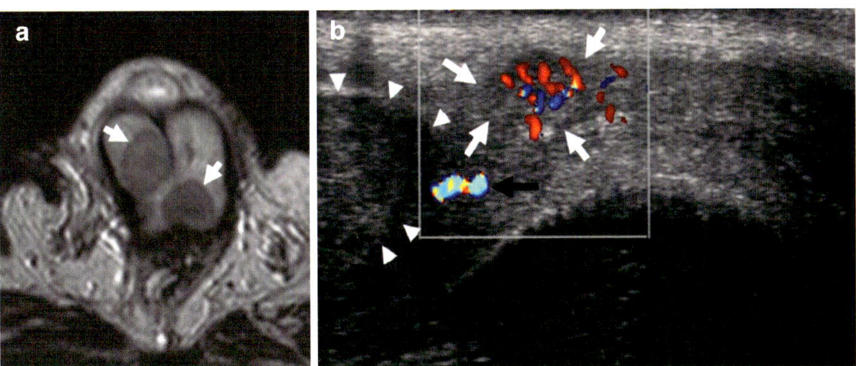

Fig. 3.7 While most T3 tumours may be adequately assessed clinically, and excision margins confirmed by frozen section, imaging helps to show these rare cases of a skip lesion in the corpus cavernosum. In (**a**), two discrete tumour foci are seen in the corpora cavernosa on T2-weighted MRI (confirmed as discontinuous on histology). In a Doppler ultrasound image from another patient (**b**), a hypervascular nodule (*white arrows*) is seen discrete from the main tumour mass (*arrowheads*). A *black arrow* marks the normal cavernosal artery. With permission from Muneer A and Horenblas S, *Textbook of Penile Cancer*, Springer International Publishing

Other Penile Tumours

Anterior urethral tumours are usually of the SCC type, with a similar appearance to other penile squamous tumour. Epithelioid sarcomas are uncommon but can mimic fibrous plaques of Peyronie's, although are not usually as low in T2 signal [16]. Benign tumours such as haemangioma, neurofibroma and lymphangioma have been described [17], and have a similar MRI appearance to elsewhere. Lymphoma is rare, usually involves the shaft and is homogenous and intermediate in signal on T1 and T2 images [18]. Melanoma is one rare tumour that can have specific MRI findings: T1 signal hyperintensity due to high protein content [19].

Finally, metastases to the penis are rare, with most of gastrointestinal or genitourinary origin (bladder, prostate, rectum, kidney, and testis—in that order) [12]. In the majority there is spread to other organs at the time of diagnosis [12], and involvement of the shaft is common, with a common presentation being obstructed voiding [20]. The imaging presentation is variable: from discrete nodules to widespread infiltration [20], with priapism more common than in primary penile tumours [12].

Nodal Staging

Full discussion of the nodal workup in penile cancer is in Chap. 8 of this book, meaning this section will focus on imaging anatomy and options. Because of the predictable route of nodal spread in penile carcinoma (with groin nodes almost always involved first [21]) there are several diagnostic paradigms for assessment. First, especially in thin patients, groin nodes may be palpable. Second, groin and pelvic nodes may be imaged using a variety of techniques (ultrasound, MRI, CT and

FDG PET, which are the focus of this chapter). Third, the nodes may be resected, either using a targeted sentinel node approach, or by superficial or radical dissection.

Nodal Anatomy & Cross-Sectional Imaging

Normal lymph nodes are usually ovoid in shape, usually with a fatty hilum, and with vessels radiating in an organised fashion from the hilum [22] (sometimes reminiscent of the vascular pattern of the kidney) (Fig. 3.8). In squamous cancer malignant nodes tend towards a round shape (hence the overarching importance of *short axis diameter*) and lose their fatty hilum [23]. Some features, such as an irregular border or fluid necrosis, are highly specific for involvement in the context of a penile cancer, but are not present in the majority [24]. One study of 32 patients (mostly with penile cancer) and 122 nodes, illustrates the problems: in 42/44 of involved nodes at least one of the following was present: long/short axis ratio < 2, absent hilum, wide cortex, or eccentric cortical widening (Fig. 3.9). The problem is that many reactive nodes had at least one of these features [25]. In the neck, Doppler studies (with measurement of resistive and pulsatility indices) can be useful [26], but experience is limited in the penis, and overall size and morphology remain the most important criteria for detecting involvement.

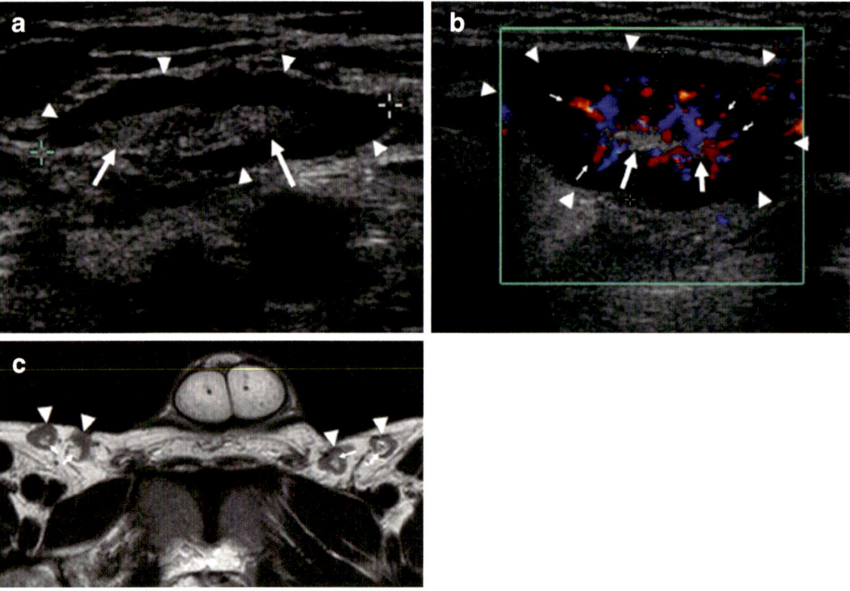

Fig. 3.8 (**a**–**c**) Features of a benign lymph node (*arrowheads*) on ultrasound, doppler ultrasound, and MRI respectively. Note the fatty hila in each case (*white arrow*). The ultrasound shows ovoid nodes with a regular cortex of uniform thickness; on doppler (**b**), small vessels radiate symmetrically from the hilum (*small white arrows*). MRI (**c**) shows nodes in *short axis*: approximately round, but with fatty hila and regular cortex. With permission from Muneer A and Horenblas S, *Textbook of Penile Cancer*, Springer International Publishing

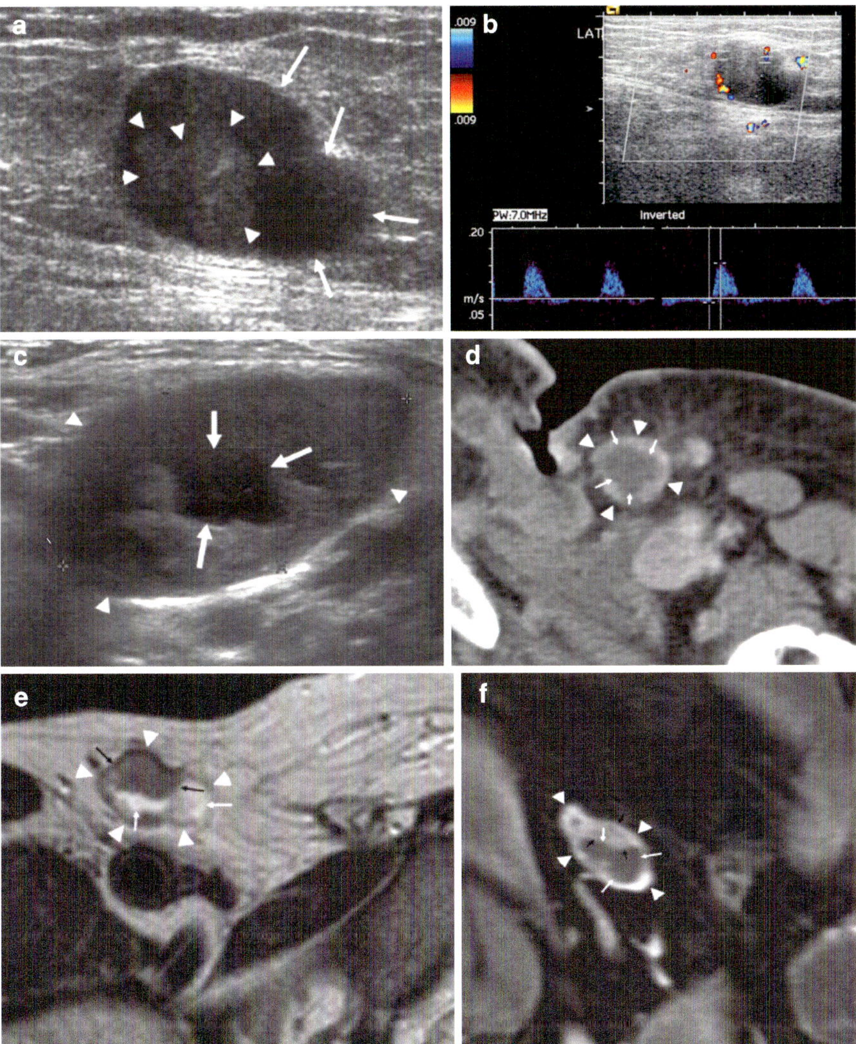

Fig. 3.9 Several features of malignant nodes. (**a**) Ultrasound shows an enlarged node with eccentric, lobulated enlargement of the cortex (*arrowheads* show the hilum, and the *arrows* the eccentric widening), and (**b**) a doppler trace of the same node showing a resistive index of 1.2. (**c**–**f**) Malignant nodes (*arrowheads*) with necrosis on ultrasound, CT, T2-weighted MRI, and postcontrast MRI (in different patients). The necrotic focus (*white arrow*, (**c**)) is nearly anechoic on ultrasound. On CT (**d**) it is of low density (close to water). (**e**) A node consisting of an eccentric nodule (*black arrow*) and fluid necrosis (*white arrow*) on a T2-weighted axial MR sequence. (**f**) A post-contrast gradient echo fat-saturated coronal sequence of the same node showing the non-enhancing necrotic component. With permission from Muneer A and Horenblas S, *Textbook of Penile Cancer*, Springer International Publishing

The most useful study assessing node size criteria specifically in penile cancer evaluated 30 patients with penile cancer using CT with the effect of different size criteria thresholds set for the groin nodes demonstrating that there is no ideal size criterion [24]. However, nodal fluid necrosis, irregular borders and adjacent infiltration were highly specific for involvement. All of these features can be seen clearly in groin nodes using CT, MRI or ultrasound (Fig. 3.9), although the latter is much less useful in the pelvis because a different probe must be used and the nodes are difficult to see well. Without these specific features the signal intensity (on MRI), density (on CT) and echogenicity (on ultrasound) of tumour within nodes is not sufficiently different to surrounding normal node to allow reliable characterisation. This limitation (small amounts of tumour do not significantly enlarge a node or change its imaging characteristics) is fundamental. A second factor is that reactive enlargement is common *at presentation* in penile cancer (occurring in 25–50% of palpable nodes [27]) but not at follow up (when palpable nodes are usually malignant [27, 28]). Conversely, although we have spent some time describing the imitations of commonly used nodal imaging techniques, there is little doubt that they (including ultrasound) are more accurate than physical examination alone [29].

Advanced Techniques: PET

SCC usually have a high glycolytic rate and show high uptake on fluorodeoxyglucose (FDG) PET [30]. Modern scanners usually have a CT or MRI capability, so that positive nodes can be co-registered with conventional cross sectional imaging, improving performance compared to each technique alone [31]. PET has potentially high sensitivity: for instance, a study in 2012 in 35 patients showed sensitivity of 88% and specificity of 98% [32], comfortably exceeding the performance of the previously mentioned size criteria.

PET may be particularly useful for pelvic node follow up: in one series of 28 hemi-pelvises, PET identified 10/11 positive cases with no false positives. However, the missed node had a deposit of 5 mm and the detected tumours were 9 mm or larger, most of which we would be detected by size criteria [33]. This raises the question: does PET have a significantly better performance than CT and MRI (enough to justify the cost and radiation burden)? A recent study confirms that it does detect more tumours in advanced disease [34], but whether it is justified in routine practice remains uncertain.

MR Lymphography

MRI usually resolves different soft tissues better than CT, but there is not reliably high contrast between tumour and normal lymph node: we still rely on size criteria, morphology and rarer but more specific findings like fluid necrosis. One way of markedly increasing this contrast is the use of superparamagnetic iron oxide particles such as ferumox-tran-10 (*Sinerem* – Guerbet, Aulnay-sous-Bois, France). If injected intravenously they are taken up by macrophages that accumulate in normal lymph nodes. The paramagnetic effect of the iron oxide then markedly reduces the T2 and T2* signal, leaving tumour deposits as foci of conspicuously high signal. This technique can detect tumour foci down to a diameter of around 2 mm [35], with on showing sensitivity (specificity) for the detection of nodal involvement in prostate cancer improved from 35% (90%) to 91% (98%) with Sinerem [36].

In a pilot study of penile cancer the results were similarly impressive (a sensitivity and specificity of 100% and 97%) [37] but the agent has not been licensed in either Europe or the USA, and is only currently available in the Netherlands [38]. However, a similar compound (Ferumoxytol) is approved for iron replacement therapy in patients with chronic kidney failure, and although not as avidly taken up by macrophages as Sinerem, has recently shown good sensitivity but lower specificity (98% and 65%) in a study of genitourinary cancers [39]. This is an area of active research, but the agent is not yet studied enough for routine clinical use.

Fine Needle Aspiration Biopsy

In palpable nodes fine needle aspiration can be a sensitive technique (detecting all 17 involved nodes in a study of 28 patients) [40] but the performance characteristics are completely different in patients without palpable nodes: here, in a study of 43 patients, Fine Needle Aspiration (FNA) of nodes suspicious on ultrasound gave a sensitivity of only 39% [41]. These findings have two clinical implications. Firstly, as a method of ruling out involvement, ultrasound +/− FNA is inadequate, although if positive is useful for triage: the patient can undergo formal inguinal node dissection without the need for sentinel node techniques [41]. Secondly, the use of ultrasound +/− FNA before sentinel node biopsy is important and effective to detect nodes that are so involved by tumour that they will not reliably take up the agents used for localisation. Such nodes are likely to be large and of abnormal morphology, and so will be detected on ultrasound in most cases, preventing a potential false negative on sentinel node localisation [41]. For this reason, the technique is an integral part of the sentinel node approach in penile cancer.

Sentinel Node Anatomy

Nodal spread of penile cancer usually involves superficial groin nodes first [21]. An initial study from 1977, showed that a sentinel node at the anterior or medial aspect of the superficial epigastric vein, medial to and above the epigastric–saphenous junction, was always involved in 15 patients with metastatic disease, and was sometimes the only site of involvement [42]. A more recent study describes it as 'the most medial inguinal node of the horizontal chain', just lateral to the pubic tubercle, but the problem is that anatomical location alone is not sufficient to identify the sentinel node: pelvic nodes have subsequently developed in several patients with negative sampling of this node [43], and a subsequent study using an 'extended' sentinel node dissection suggested that even this technique might miss a quarter of involved groins and could not be recommended [44]. The technique and

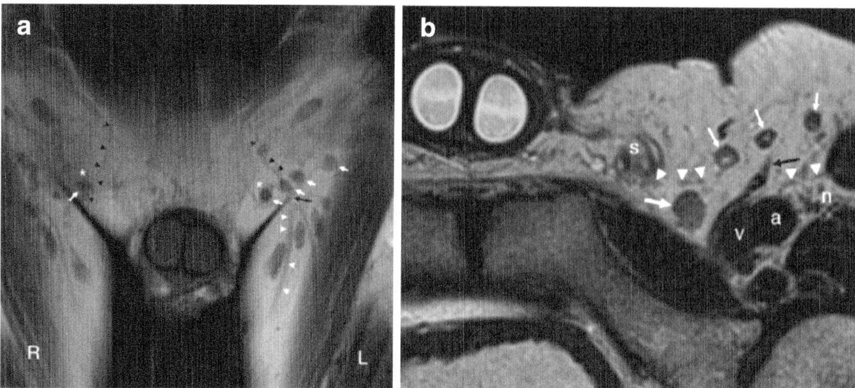

Fig. 3.10 (**a**) Thick-slab T1 spin echo coronal image of the superficial inguinal nodes. The horizontal group is shown by the *white arrows*: the most medial (*asterisk*) is defined as the 'sentinel' node. *Black arrowheads* mark the superficial epigastric vein; note that on the left the sentinel node lies medial to the superficial epigastric vein, but on the right is anterior to it. *White arrowheads* mark the long saphenous vein and the *black arrow* the junction between the superficial epigastric and long saphenous veins. (**b**) Axial T2-weighted image of the groin in a patient scanned because of a penile prosthesis. Note the horizontal chain of the superficial nodes (*small white arrows*, each with a fatty hilum). They lie superficial to the fascia lata (*white arrowheads*). The saphenous vein (*black arrow*) passes through the cribriform fascia (lying in the oval defect of the fascia lata) to join the femoral vein (*v*). The femoral artery is marked a, the femoral nerve *n*, and the spermatic cord *s*. The *larger white arrow* shows a deep inguinal node medial to the femoral vein. With permission from Muneer A and Horenblas S, *Textbook of Penile Cancer*, Springer International Publishing

performance of sentinel node biopsy is discussed in more detail in Chap. 8 but the anatomy is described here because when imaging the groins (whether by ultrasound, CT or MRI) it is useful to know the most likely site of nodal involvement (Fig. 3.10).

Imaging of Metastases

Metastatic disease is present in only 3% of patients at presentation, with the commonest sites lung, liver, retroperitoneum and bone [45]. Because prognosis is poor, the focus of initial screening investigation is not on the detection of metastatic disease, and the EAU 2018 guidelines only recommend CT of abdomen and pelvis (with either chest X ray or CT) in the presence of nodal involvement, with a bone scan in the case of bone metastases (although whole body MRI may be more sensitive [46] and is an alternative). Alternatively, complete staging can be achieved by combined PET/CT [30].

EAU Guidelines and Protocols for Staging and Follow Up

The 2018 EAU guidelines [1] give an approach for the investigation and follow up of penile cancer, briefly summarised here.

Initial staging can be divided into the TNM classification:

T: Recent evidence on the utility of ultrasound with artificial erection (and potential superiority to MRI) mean that now either MRI or ultrasound are given a 'weak' rating: to be used in selected cases rather than routinely. For some time some groups have advocated MRI for all cases of suspected penile cancer, but this is not part of the guidelines [7].

N: In cases of impalpable nodes with a low-risk primary tumour (Tis, Ta G1, potentially T1G1), clinical surveillance is adequate. Some authors sample cases of pT1 G1 disease [27] and nomograms can be used to triage sampling according to risk based on clinical and pathological findings [47], though this is not part of the guidelines and is not genrally used in clinical practice.

For higher risk patients with impalpable nodes, 'invasive nodal sampling' is advised. Dynamic sentinel node sampling is the gold standard. However, modified inguinal lymphadenectomy can be used as an alternative technique in cases where DSNB is not available.

With palpable nodes the likelihood of involvement is high, and time should not be wasted waiting for possible infection to settle. The nodes should either be assessed with ultrasound +/− FNA or a superficial modified inguinal node dissection performed (with frozen section of the lymph node packet to confirm involvement before the complete dissection is performed). In this case, pelvic CT 'can provide staging information' (it is likely that this is routine in most centres), with PET/CT able to 'identify additional metastases'.

M: All cases of node positive disease should undergo CT of the abdomen and pelvis. With modern CT it is easier and more accurate to include the chest in the scan than perform a plain CXR, and this is our routine practice. A bone can is recommended 'with systemic disease or relevant symptom'. PET/CT is an alternative to MRI/CT + bone scan. Whole body MRI is not yet mentioned.

Protocols for Follow Up

For the primary tumour, the EAU recommends clinical follow up rather than imaging in its 2018 guidelines. For the inguinal nodes, follow up recommendations depend on initial nodal status. With node negative disease in intermediate to high-risk tumours, clinical examination every 3 months for a year, and then annually to 5 years. Ultrasound +/− FNA 'optional'. With initially node positive disease, clinical examination every 3 months for a year, and then 6 monthly to 5 years. Ultrasound +/− FNA are 'optional', as are CT and MRI. At the authors' institution ultrasound is used routinely, both for node positive and intermediate to high-risk node negative patients.

Future Directions

The recent data on the performance of ultrasound in local staging [14] may result in a move to stage by ultrasound in some centres, although the technique remains operator-dependent, and further studies are awaited.

For nodal staging PET/CT is fundamentally limited and gives a relatively high radiation dose. Iron oxide particles have the *potential* to significantly improve assessment, but have been in the 'potential' category for some time, and do potentially require two visits, intravenous administration and experienced radiologists [39].

For metastatic disease it is likely that whole body MRI will supersede bone scans [46], although PET/CT remains an alternative with good performance: comparisons of the two techniques are starting to emerge, but not yet in penile cancer.

Key Points

- Staging the primary tumour through imaging before operation is not always indicated in penile cancer.
- Ultrasound has comparable efficacy to MRI for staging the local tumour and groin lymph nodes.
- Ultrasound +/− FNA are an important part of sentinel node techniques, to avoid missing involved nodes that do not take up tracer.
- Nodal staging with any modality (ultrasound, CT, MRI, PET) is not highly accurate, although there are some specific signs of nodal involvement (in particular, necrosis).
- Ultrasound and FNA have a low sensitivity for detecting nodal involvement in clinically negative groins and cannot substitute for groin dissection or sentinel node biopsy.

Revision Questions

Multiple Choice Questions

1. Concerning the use of MRI for staging penile cancer, which of these is true
   A. Contrast enhancement is essential for optimum diagnostic performance.
   B. Guidelines recommend the use of MRI / ultrasound in all cases
   C. MRI has demonstrably superior performance to ultrasound.
   D. None of the above
2. Which of these is a useful feature of lymph nodes involved with tumour?
   A. The appearance of fluid within the node.
   B. A long axis diameter of >1 cm
   C. A fatty hilum
   D. None of the above

3. Ultrasound +/− FNA before surgery
   A. Has a sufficient sensitivity to be used for nodal staging
   B. Is indicated before techniques using tracer or dye to identify the sentinel node
   C. Cannot be used to triage patients with involved nodes to radical groin dissection
   D. None of the above
4. Concerning the EAU 2018 guidelines for penile cancer:
   A. All patients should be followed up with ultrasound of the groins for 5 years.
   B. Sentinel node biopsy or groin dissection are indicated in all patients with proven tumour, unless there are contraindications
   C. All patients should undergo CT of chest, abdomen and pelvis.
   D. None of the above.

Viva Cases

Case 1

A patient you have evaluated in clinic has after biopsy been confirmed to have penile cancer.

A. Should you routinely perform local staging of penile cancer before surgery?

Case 2

Following local staging a patient in clinic requires further evaluation for nodal and metastatic spread.

A. What is the most sensitive single imaging technique for detecting nodal and metastatic disease in high grade tumours, and should it be used routinely?

Answers

Multiple Choice Questions

1. **D.** Ultrasound and MRI are of similar efficacy according to recent high-quality data. Contrast helps little. Routine staging is not necessary.
2. **A.** The short axis measurement is key in lymph nodes. Fatty hilum is a benign feature. Fluid, however, is highly specific for involvement in the context of SCC.
3. **B.** US +/− FNA is specific but not sensitive. This means that when positive it can be used to triage patients to radical node dissection. However, it is not sensitive enough to be used for staging. Because a positive finding is a useful result (and prevents false negative tracer uptake from bulky nodal involvement) it is useful before sentinel node biopsy.

4. **A.** Although many centres would perform CT of chest, abdomen and pelvis for any penile cancer, this is not yet part of the guidelines. Sentinel node sampling is not indicated for low risk primary tumours. However, 5 year follow up of the groins is in the recommendations for all patients.

Viva Cases
Case 1

A. No, in 2018 EAU guidelines imaging is not indicated routinely for local staging. In many cases clinical examination is accurate, and in addition the operative findings are likely to be the gold standard for determining the extent of the resection. Imaging can be useful for 'problem solving' or patient counselling about the likely extent of resection but should be reserved for selected cases.

Case 2

A. CT/PET is the only single technique that can detect metastases in lymph nodes, chest and bone with high sensitivity. MRI (including whole body MRI) does not have a high sensitivity in the chest, and standard contrast-enhanced CT has a lower sensitivity than CT/PET. However, routine use is probably not indicated because (a) it has a high dose technique, (b) it is expensive, and (c) early detection of metastatic (as opposed to nodal) disease may not necessarily lead to clinical benefit.

Test your learning and check your understanding of this book's contents: use the "Springer Nature Flashcards" app to access questions using ▸ https://sn.pub/1r7Om8. To use the app, please follow the instructions in chapter 1.

References

1. Hakenberg OW, Compérat E, Minhas ES, Necchi A, Pretzel C, Watkin N. European Association of Urology guidelines: penile cancer. The Netherlands: EAU Guidelines Office; 2021. [Available from: https://uroweb.org/guideline/penile-cancer]
2. Krishna S, Shanbhogue K, Schieda N, Morbeck F, Hadas B, Kulkarni G, et al. Role of MRI in staging of penile cancer. J Magn Reson Imaging. 2020;51(6):1612–29.
3. Pretorius ES, Siegelman ES, Ramchandani P, Banner MP. MR imaging of the penis. Radiographics. 2001;21(suppl_1):S283–S98.
4. Kirkham A. MRI of the penis. Br J Radiol. 2012;85. Spec No 1:S86-93.
5. Hanchanale V, Yeo L, Subedi N, Smith J, Wah T, Harnden P, et al. The accuracy of magnetic resonance imaging (MRI) in predicting the invasion of the tunica albuginea and the urethra during the primary staging of penile cancer. BJU Int. 2016;117(3):439–43.
6. Barua SK, Kaman PK, Baruah SJ, Rajeev TP, Bagchi PK, Sarma D, et al. Role of diffusion-weighted magnetic resonance imaging (DWMRI) in assessment of primary penile tumor characteristics and its correlations with inguinal lymph node metastasis: a prospective study. World J Oncol. 2018;9(5–6):145–50.

7. Kochhar R, Taylor B, Sangar V. Imaging in primary penile cancer: current status and future directions. Eur Radiol. 2010;20(1):36–47.
8. Ghosh P, Chandra A, Mukhopadhyay S, Chatterjee A, Lingegowda D, Gehani A, et al. Accuracy of MRI without intracavernosal prostaglandin E1 injection in staging, preoperative evaluation, and operative planning of penile cancer. Abdom Radiol (NY). 2021;46(10):4984–94.
9. Scardino E, Villa G, Bonomo G, Matei DV, Verweij F, Rocco B, et al. Magnetic resonance imaging combined with artificial erection for local staging of penile cancer. Urology. 2004;63(6):1158–62.
10. Linet OI, Ogrinc FG. Efficacy and safety of intracavernosal alprostadil in men with erectile dysfunction. The Alprostadil Study Group. N Engl J Med. 1996;334(14):873–7.
11. Muruve N, Hosking DH. Intracorporeal phenylephrine in the treatment of priapism. J Urol. 1996;155(1):141–3.
12. Chan PT, Begin LR, Arnold D, Jacobson SA, Corcos J, Brock GB. Priapism secondary to penile metastasis: a report of two cases and a review of the literature. J Surg Oncol. 1998;68(1):51–9.
13. Minhas S, Kayes O, Hegarty P, Kumar P, Freeman A, Ralph D. What surgical resection margins are required to achieve oncological control in men with primary penile cancer? BJU Int. 2005;96(7):1040–3.
14. Bozzini G, Provenzano M, Romero Otero J, Margreiter M, Garcia Cruz E, Osmolorskij B, et al. Role of Penile Doppler US in the preoperative assessment of penile squamous cell carcinoma patients: results from a large prospective Multicenter European Study. Urology. 2016;90:131–5.
15. Lont AP, Besnard AP, Gallee MP, van Tinteren H, Horenblas S. A comparison of physical examination and imaging in determining the extent of primary penile carcinoma. BJU Int. 2003;91(6):493–5.
16. Sirikci A, Bayram M, Demirci M, Bakir K, Sarica K. Penile epithelioid sarcoma: MR imaging findings. Eur Radiol. 1999;9(8):1593–5.
17. Dehner LP, Smith BH. Soft tissue tumors of the penis. A clinicopathologic study of 46 cases. Cancer. 1970;25(6):1431–47.
18. Chiang KH, Chang PY, Lee SK, Yen PS, Ling CM, Lin CC, et al. MR findings of penile lymphoma. Br J Radiol. 2006;79(942):526–8.
19. Gaviani P, Mullins ME, Braga TA, Hedley-Whyte ET, Halpern EF, Schaefer PS, et al. Improved detection of metastatic melanoma by T2*-weighted imaging. AJNR Am J Neuroradiol. 2006;27(3):605–8.
20. Lau TN, Wakeley CJ, Goddard P. Magnetic resonance imaging of penile metastases: a report on five cases. Australas Radiol. 1999;43(3):378–81.
21. Leijte JA, Kirrander P, Antonini N, Windahl T, Horenblas S. Recurrence patterns of squamous cell carcinoma of the penis: recommendations for follow-up based on a two-centre analysis of 700 patients. Eur Urol. 2008;54(1):161–8.
22. Restrepo R, Oneto J, Lopez K, Kukreja K. Head and neck lymph nodes in children: the spectrum from normal to abnormal. Pediatr Radiol. 2009;39(8):836–46.
23. Ahuja AT, Ying M. Sonographic evaluation of cervical lymph nodes. AJR Am J Roentgenol. 2005;184(5):1691–9.
24. Graafland NM, Teertstra HJ, Besnard AP, van Boven HH, Horenblas S. Identification of high risk pathological node positive penile carcinoma: value of preoperative computerized tomography imaging. J Urol. 2011;185(3):881–7.
25. Krishna RP, Sistla SC, Smile R, Krishnan R. Sonography: an underutilized diagnostic tool in the assessment of metastatic groin nodes. J Clin Ultrasound. 2008;36(4):212–7.
26. Steinkamp HJ, Maurer J, Cornehl M, Knobber D, Hettwer H, Felix R. Recurrent cervical lymphadenopathy: differential diagnosis with color-duplex sonography. Eur Arch Otorhinolaryngol. 1994;251(7):404–9.
27. Hughes B, Leijte J, Shabbir M, Watkin N, Horenblas S. Non-invasive and minimally invasive staging of regional lymph nodes in penile cancer. World J Urol. 2009;27(2):197–203.
28. Ornellas AA, Seixas AL, Marota A, Wisnescky A, Campos F, de Moraes JR. Surgical treatment of invasive squamous cell carcinoma of the penis: retrospective analysis of 350 cases. J Urol. 1994;151(5):1244–9.

29. Leone A, Diorio GJ, Pettaway C, Master V, Spiess PE. Contemporary management of patients with penile cancer and lymph node metastasis. Nat Rev Urol. 2017;14(6):335–47.
30. Scher B, Seitz M, Reiser M, Hungerhuber E, Hahn K, Tiling R, et al. 18F-FDG PET/CT for staging of penile cancer. J Nucl Med. 2005;46(9):1460–5.
31. Veit P, Ruehm S, Kuehl H, Stergar H, Mueller S, Bockisch A, et al. Lymph node staging with dual-modality PET/CT: enhancing the diagnostic accuracy in oncology. Eur J Radiol. 2006;58(3):383–9.
32. Schlenker B, Scher B, Tiling R, Siegert S, Hungerhuber E, Gratzke C, et al. Detection of inguinal lymph node involvement in penile squamous cell carcinoma by 18F-fluorodeoxyglucose PET/CT: a prospective single-center study. Urol Oncol. 2012;30(1):55–9.
33. Graafland NM, Leijte JA, Valdes Olmos RA, Hoefnagel CA, Teertstra HJ, Horenblas S. Scanning with 18F-FDG-PET/CT for detection of pelvic nodal involvement in inguinal node-positive penile carcinoma. Eur Urol. 2009;56(2):339–45.
34. Zhang S, Li W, Liang F. Clinical value of fluorine-18 2-fluoro-2-deoxy-D-glucose positron emission tomography/computed tomography in penile cancer. Oncotarget. 2016;7(30):48600–6.
35. Harisinghani MG, Saksena M, Ross RW, Tabatabaei S, Dahl D, McDougal S, et al. A pilot study of lymphotrophic nanoparticle-enhanced magnetic resonance imaging technique in early stage testicular cancer: a new method for noninvasive lymph node evaluation. Urology. 2005;66(5):1066–71.
36. Harisinghani MG, Barentsz J, Hahn PF, Deserno WM, Tabatabaei S, van de Kaa CH, et al. Noninvasive detection of clinically occult lymph-node metastases in prostate cancer. N Engl J Med. 2003;348(25):2491–9.
37. Tabatabaei S, Harisinghani M, McDougal WS. Regional lymph node staging using lymphotropic nanoparticle enhanced magnetic resonance imaging with ferumoxtran-10 in patients with penile cancer. J Urol. 2005;174(3):923–7. discussion 7
38. Fortuin AS, Bruggemann R, van der Linden J, Panfilov I, Israel B, Scheenen TWJ, et al. Ultra-small superparamagnetic iron oxides for metastatic lymph node detection: back on the block. Wiley Interdiscip Rev Nanomed Nanobiotechnol. 2018;10:1.
39. Turkbey B, Czarniecki M, Shih JH, Harmon SA, Agarwal PK, Apolo AB, et al. Ferumoxytol-enhanced MR lymphography for detection of metastatic lymph nodes in genitourinary malignancies: a prospective study. AJR Am J Roentgenol. 2020;214(1):105–13.
40. Senthil Kumar MP, Ananthakrishnan N, Prema V. Predicting regional lymph node metastasis in carcinoma of the penis: a comparison between fine-needle aspiration cytology, sentinel lymph node biopsy and medial inguinal lymph node biopsy. Br J Urol. 1998;81(3):453–7.
41. Kroon BK, Horenblas S, Deurloo EE, Nieweg OE, Teertstra HJ. Ultrasonography-guided fine-needle aspiration cytology before sentinel node biopsy in patients with penile carcinoma. BJU Int. 2005;95(4):517–21.
42. Cabanas RM. An approach for the treatment of penile carcinoma. Cancer. 1977;39(2):456–66.
43. Wespes E, Simon J, Schulman CC. Cabanas approach: is sentinel node biopsy reliable for staging penile carcinoma? Urology. 1986;28(4):278–9.
44. Pettaway CA, Pisters LL, Dinney CP, Jularbal F, Swanson DA, von Eschenbach AC, et al. Sentinel lymph node dissection for penile carcinoma: the M. D. Anderson Cancer Center experience. J Urol. 1995;154(6):1999–2003.
45. Rippentrop JM, Joslyn SA, Konety BR. Squamous cell carcinoma of the penis: evaluation of data from the surveillance, epidemiology, and end results program. Cancer. 2004;101(6):1357–63.
46. Morone M, Bali MA, Tunariu N, Messiou C, Blackledge M, Grazioli L, et al. Whole-body MRI: current applications in oncology. AJR Am J Roentgenol. 2017;209(6):W336–W49.
47. Ficarra V, Zattoni F, Artibani W, Fandella A, Martignoni G, Novara G, et al. Nomogram predictive of pathological inguinal lymph node involvement in patients with squamous cell carcinoma of the penis. J Urol. 2006;175(5):1700–4. discussion 4-5.

Diagnosing and Staging Patients with Penile Cancer

4

Alice Yu, Jad Chahoud, Jasreman Dhillon, and Philippe E. Spiess

Learning Objectives
After reading this chapter you will be able to:

- Conduct a comprehensive clinical assessment of patients presenting with possible penile cancer, including history and examination
- Review common histological subtypes of penile cancer and their relevance for staging of the disease
- Describe the widely utilised TNM staging classifications of penile cancer
- Apply diagnostic pathways for accurate staging of disease

History and Physical Exam

Penile cancer is relatively rare in North America and Europe (<1% of all malignant neoplasms), however, remains a health concern in many African, South American, and Asian countries [1]. It occurs primarily in older men with a peak incidence in the sixth decade [2]. Risk factors for penile cancer are discussed in detail in Chap. 1 and in summary include lack of neonatal circumcision, chronic inflammation, phimosis, lichen sclerosus, tobacco use, obesity, poor hygiene, exposure to UV radiation, history of sexually transmitted diseases, and human papillomavirus (HPV) infection [1, 3]. It has been estimated that 45–80% of penile cancers are related to HPV infection, particularly subtypes 6, 16 and 18 [4].

A. Yu · J. Chahoud · P. E. Spiess (✉)
Department of Genitourinary Oncology, H. Lee Moffitt Cancer Center, Tampa, FL, USA
e-mail: philippe.spiess@moffitt.org

J. Dhillon
Department of Pathology, H. Lee Moffitt Cancer Center, Tampa, FL, USA

O. Brunckhorst et al. (eds.), *Penile Cancer – A Practical Guide*, Management of Urology, https://doi.org/10.1007/978-3-031-32681-3_4

Penile cancer can arise anywhere on the penis but occurs most commonly on the glans (48%) and prepuce (21%) [5]. These lesions can appear papillary, nodular, ulcerative, flat (Fig. 4.1) or fungating. Penile Intraepithelial neoplasia (PeIN) is referred eponymously as Erythroplasia of Queyrat when it appears on the glans or inner prepuce and Bowen's Disease when it appears on the penile shaft. PeIN can appear as a red, velvety, well-marginated flat lesion.

If left untreated, penile cancer can become ulcerative and/or infected. A non-healing lesion of the penis should raise suspicion for a malignant process and a biopsy should be considered. Penile cancer is often asymptomatic although pain, discharge and bleeding can be seen in advanced cases with extensive local tissue destruction. Urinary symptoms and obstruction are less common though it can occur in locally advanced disease. Patients with metastatic spread may also experience constitutional symptoms such as fatigue, poor appetite, and weight loss.

On physical examination, clinicians should note the size, morphology, location, fixation to adjacent structures, and involvement of the corpora cavernosum and spongiosa. In uncircumcised men, the lesion can be hidden under the prepuce due to the presence of a phimosis and therefore careful palpation and retraction of the prepuce is necessary. In addition, inspection of the base of the penis and scrotum for tumour extension and additional lesions should be performed.

Palpation of the inguinal area is important to assess for lymphadenopathy which should record the number of palpable lymph nodes, laterality, approximate size, consistency (hard vs. rubbery) and whether lymph nodes are mobile or fixed. It is important to differentiate whether the tumour is fixed to deeper structures or the overlying skin as this will impact on whether the tumour is resectable and the type of surgical reconstruction can be performed.

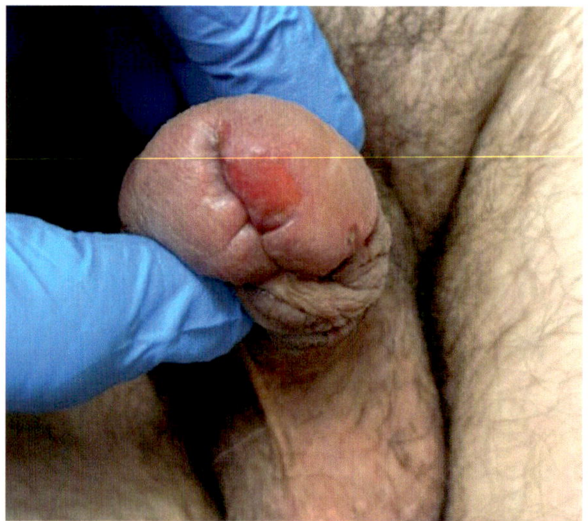

Fig. 4.1 Penile squamous cell carcinoma, flat lesion, affecting the meatus [6]

Table 4.1 Differential diagnosis of penile lesion

Inflammatory conditions	Infectious conditions	Malignancy
• Genital psoriasis • Angiokeratomas • Lichen planus • Lichen sclerosus	• Primary syphilis • Herpes • Granuloma inguinale • Tuberculosis • Condyloma acuminatum	• Squamous cell carcinoma • Melanoma • Basal cell carcinoma • Kaposi sarcoma • Other penile sarcomas • Extramammary Paget's disease • Urethral carcinoma • Metastasis

Biopsy and Pathology

Various benign penile lesions must be considered in the differential diagnosis of a penile lesion (Table 4.1).

A biopsy of the primary lesion is mandatory to confirm the diagnosis of penile carcinoma and to determine tumour characteristics, such as the depth of invasion, histologic grade, presence of lymphovascular invasion (LVI) and perineural invasion (PNI). These pathologic features are important for staging and risk stratification. Biopsy can be performed as a separate procedure or at the time of definitive surgical treatment with frozen-section confirmation. Full discussion on penile cancer pathology including histological features, classifications of penile SCC, grading and example pathology slides can be found within Chap. 2 of this textbook.

Staging of Penile Cancer

The AJCC TNM (tumour, node, and metastasis) staging system for penile cancer, 8th ed., 2017 is described in Tables 4.2 and 4.3 [7].

Table 4.2 The AJCC TNM (tumour, node, and metastasis) staging system for penile cancer, 8th ed., 2017

Tx	Primary tumour cannot be assessed
T0	No evidence of primary tumour
Tis	Carcinoma *in situ* (penile intraepithelial neoplasia [PeIN])
Ta	Non-invasive localized squamous cell carcinoma
T1	Glans: Tumour invades lamina propria Foreskin: Tumour invades dermis, lamina propria, or dartos fascia Shaft: Tumour invades connective tissue between epidermis and corpora regardless of location All sites with or without lymphovascular invasion or perineural invasion and is or is not high grade
T1a	Tumour is without lymphovascular invasion or perineural invasion and is not high grade (i.e., grade 3 or sarcomatoid)
T1b	Tumour exhibits lymphovascular invasion and/or perineural invasion or is high grade (i.e., grade 3 or sarcomatoid)
T2	Tumour invades into corpus spongiosum (either glans or ventral shaft) with or without urethral invasion
T3	Tumour invades into corpora cavernosa (including tunica albuginea) with or without urethral invasion
T4	Tumour invades into adjacent structures (i.e., scrotum, prostate, pubic bone)
cNX	Regional lymph nodes cannot be assessed
cN0	No palpable or visibly enlarged inguinal lymph nodes
cN1	Palpable mobile unilateral inguinal lymph node
cN2	Palpable mobile ≥2 unilateral inguinal nodes or bilateral inguinal lymph nodes
cN3	Palpable fixed inguinal nodal mass or pelvic lymphadenopathy unilateral or bilateral
pNX	Lymph node metastasis cannot be established
pN0	No lymph node metastasis
pN1	≤2 unilateral inguinal metastases, no ENE
pN2	≥3 unilateral inguinal metastases or bilateral metastases
pN3	ENE of lymph node metastases or pelvic lymph node metastases, no ENE
M0	No distant metastasis
M1	Distant metastasis present

Table 4.3 AJCC anatomic stage/prognostic groups

	T	N	M
Stage 0is	Tis	N0	M0
Stage 0a	Ta	N0	M0
Stage I	T1a	N0	M0
Stage IIA	T1b	N0	M0
	T2	N0	M0
Stage IIB	T3	N0	M0
Stage IIIA	T1–3	N1	M0
Stage IIIB	T1–3	N3	M0
Stage IV	T4	Any N	M0
	Any T	N3	M0
	Any T	Any N	M1

Staging of the Primary Tumour

Staging of the primary tumour is important for risk stratification and determining treatment options. Often, physical examination alone is sufficient to establish the clinical stage, however, this can be more challenging in small, superficial tumours. It has been suggested that physical examination under-stages in 10% and over-stages in 16% of cases when compared to the final surgical pathology [8].

As discussed in Chap. 3, imaging can be added as an adjunct, especially when organ-sparing techniques are being considered. For local staging, MRI is often the modality of choice with CT lacking the soft tissue contrast resolution to distinguish penile cancer from normal anatomic structures. Ultrasound can also be considered, though this is variable across centres according to local expertise with some studies showing poorer higher sensitivity and specificity.

Staging of Inguinal Lymph Nodes

Penile lymphangiographic studies have demonstrated a predictable pattern of lymphatic drainage that goes from the penis to the superficial inguinal lymph nodes (ILNs) and then to the deep inguinal (deep to the fascia lata) followed by drainage to the pelvic lymph nodes [9]. Lymphatic drainage is bilateral to both inguinal regions with multiple cross connections at each level therefore surgical staging should always be performed bilaterally.

Lymph node metastasis is the most important prognostic factor for penile cancer [10–12] and careful evaluation of the groins and pelvis are essential components of penile cancer workup which is discussed in Chap. 8. Figure 4.2 provides a summary on the decision to perform invasive ILN staging depending on a variety of factors including presence of palpable inguinal lymph nodes and risk of occult metastasis based on stage of the primary tumour.

Palpable Lymph Nodes

Palpable ILNs are highly indicative of lymph node metastasis. In patients with palpable inguinal lymphadenopathy, additional cross-sectional imaging of the chest, abdomen and pelvis should be performed to rule out distant metastasis. Ultrasound guided fine needle aspiration (FNAC) helps to confirm diagnosis. If FNAC is positive, the patient should undergo radical inguinal node dissection. The EAU guidelines add that staging with PET/CT is also acceptable [13]. If distant metastasis is not detected, additional staging varies depending on the bulkiness of the lymph nodes and the risk of metastasis based on the primary lesion (Fig. 4.2).

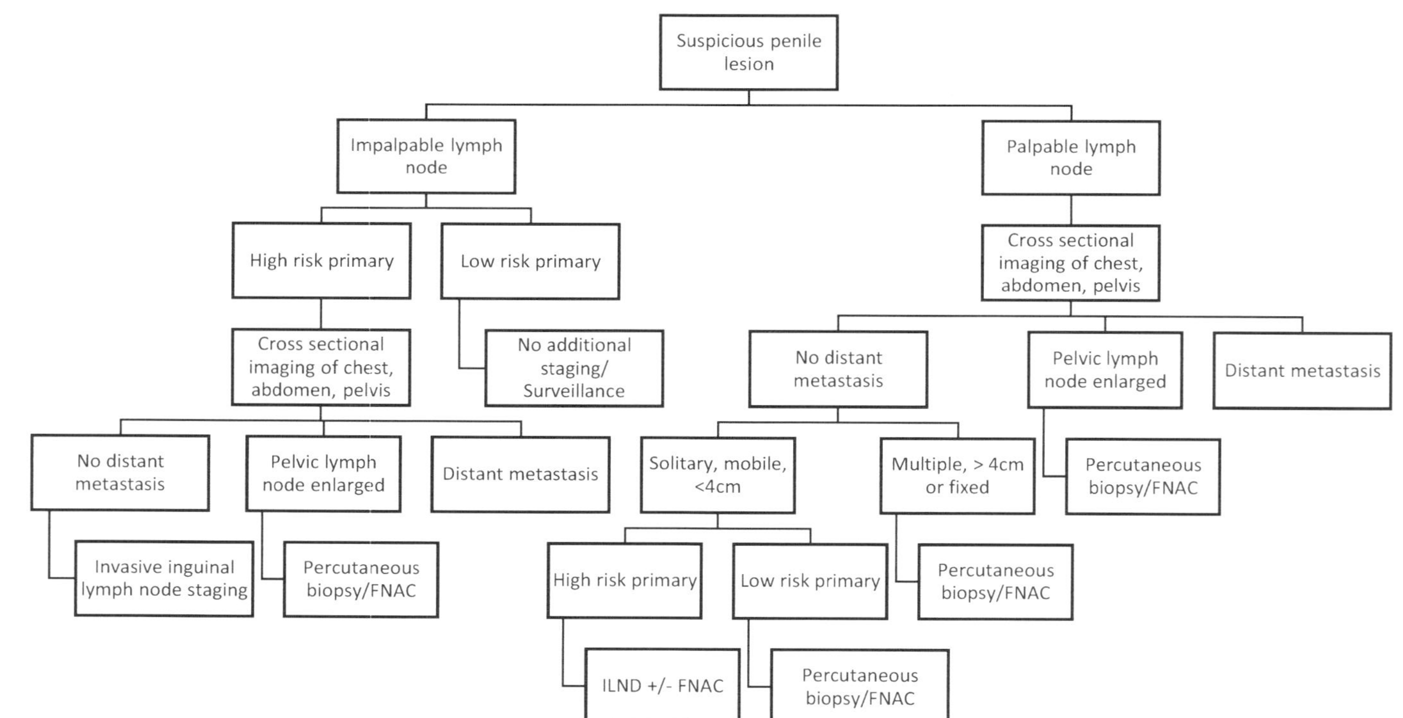

Fig. 4.2 Summary of metastatic work up for penile cancer

In the United States, the National Comprehensive Cancer Network (NCCN) guidelines recommend that in patients with unilateral palpable lymph nodes that are mobile and < 4 cm, percutaneous ILN biopsy should be performed if no high-risk features are present in the primary penile lesion [14]. A negative biopsy can be followed by surveillance or excisional biopsy. Patients with a positive biopsy should undergo treatment.

In contrast, if the primary lesion is high risk, then patients with a unilateral, <4 cm, mobile ILN should proceed to treatment without biopsy. These patients should directly undergo inguinal lymph node dissection (ILND) which may be both diagnostic and potentially curative.

Patients with large (>4 cm), bilateral or fixed ILNs should undergo ultrasound guided fine needle aspiration (FNAC) or percutaneous biopsy for diagnosis. If FNAC or biopsy is positive, they may require radical inguinal lymph node dissection +/− pedicled flap or systemic treatment as discussed in Chap. 9.

The practice in Europe is similar though ultrasound guided FNAC is more utilised whereas percutaneous biopsy is less frequently performed. The EAU advocates for surgical removal of palpable, resectable, inguinal lymph nodes and if positive on frozen section, radical inguinal lymphadenectomy should be performed. In patients with fixed inguinal lymph nodes, histologic verification by biopsy is not required if diagnosis is unequivocal.

Non-palpable Lymph Nodes

Patients with ≥ T1G2 in the primary tumour are at high risk of lymphatic metastasis with a risk of micro-metastasis of approximately 25% [15]. Imaging is not useful for staging since it often fails to detect metastasis <10 mm [16]. Indication for invasive staging should be guided by pathology of the primary tumour and patient with intermediate (G2pT1) or high-risk disease (≥ G3pT1) should be offered Invasive lymph node staging with sentinel node biopsy (gold standard) or modified lymph node dissection, both discussed in further detail in Chap. 8.

In patients where the inguinal region is difficult to assess due to reasons such as obesity or previous surgery, MRI is an option. Positron emission tomography (PET) with ^{18}F-fluorodeoxyglucose (FDG) is based on cellular uptake of glucose and FDG, which is elevated in malignant cells and other tissues with an elevated glycolytic rate [17]. It is particularly useful for the diagnosis of distant metastasis in the setting of cN+ disease, however, the sensitivity of detecting metastasis with cN0 is modest as demonstrated by multiple studies [18–20]. A 2012, meta-analysis including seven studies, demonstrated a pooled sensitivity per groin for FDG-PET/CT in cN0 patients reported as 56.5% (95% CI, 34.5%–76.8%) [21]. Based on this, FDG-PET/CT is not recommended for routine staging of cN0 tumours, and surgical staging remains a necessity to identify small inguinal lymph node metastases for staging of patients with cN0 tumours with high-risk features.

The European Association of Urology (EAU) also recommends inguinal ultrasound (7.5 MHz) in obese patients whom palpation is unreliable. This is based on a publication in 2008 that reported relatively high specificity of ultrasound in detection of metastatic groin lymph nodes. Suspicious features include longitudinal/transverse diameter ratio < 2 and absence of lymph node hilum [22].

Staging for Metastasis

Staging for pelvic metastasis should be performed in patients with palpable inguinal lymph nodes or if distant metastasis is suspected. In patients with ILN metastasis, many will have pelvic lymph node (PLN) involvement. More specifically, if 2–3 ILNs are positive, there is a 23% chance of PLN disease. If 3 or more ILNs are involved, this probability increases to 56% [23]. Additional independent predictors of PLN metastasis include the diameter of the ILN metastasis and presence of extracapsular extension [24]

An abdominopelvic CT scan can be used to assess for pelvic and/or retroperitoneal lymphadenopathy as well as distant intra-abdominal metastasis. Thoracic CT should be obtained for additional staging. PET/CT has shown high sensitivity and specificity (91% and 100%, respectively) for metastatic pelvic lymph nodes in patients with proven inguinal metastasis [16]

Key Points

- Penile cancer is relatively rare in North America and Europe. However, it is still a significant health concern in other parts of the world
- Several environmental and personal risk factors exist
- Penile cancers can present as asymptomatic lesions. Diagnosis involves taking a history, careful physical exam, and biopsy
- Stage, grade, presence of LVI and PNI in the primary tumour are important prognostic factors used for staging and risk stratification

Revision Questions

Multiple Choice Questions

1. Which of the following is not a typical risk factor for penile cancer?
   A. Tobacco use
   B. Chronic inflammation

   C. Circumcision
   D. Lichen sclerosus

2. Which of the following is most commonly associated with penile carcinoma?
   A. Herpes zoster
   B. BK virus
   C. HPV 8 and 11
   D. HPV 16 and 18

3. Which of the following conditions is malignant?
   A. Angiokeratoma
   B. Extramammary Paget disease
   C. Granuloma inguinale
   D. Condyloma acuminatum

4. Which of the following is not a factor included in penile cancer staging?
   A. Size of the penile tumour
   B. Presence of LVI
   C. Presence of PNI
   D. Sarcomatoid histology

5. A 70-year-old man has a 2 cm squamous cell carcinoma on the penile shaft underwent total penectomy with bilateral inguinal lymph node dissection. The penile tumour showed invasion into the corpus spongiosum and urethra with no involvement of the corpora cavernosa. He has 2/10 positive lymph nodes on the right, largest measuring 1 cm and 0/10 positive lymph nodes on the left. There was no extranodal extension. PET scan showed no distant metastasis. What is the stage of his disease?
   A. pT2N1M0
   B. pT3N1M0
   C. pT2N2M0
   D. pT3N2M0

6. A 60-year-old man presents to your office with a 2 cm papillary lesion on the prepuce no palpable lymph nodes. He undergoes circumcision and final surgical pathology reveals squamous cell carcinoma, pT1 Grade 3 with LVI. Imaging of the abdomen and pelvis are negative. Which of the following therapies are indication at this stage?
   A. Surveillance
   B. Biopsy of the right inguinal lymph node
   C. Bilateral inguinal lymph node dissection

7. A 75 M with a large penile lesion underwent partial penectomy. Final pathology was SCC pT3. He has 1.5 cm right inguinal lymph node that is palpable and mobile. What is the next step in management?
   A. Right inguinal lymph node dissection
   B. Bilateral inguinal lymph node dissection
   C. Percutaneous biopsy of the inguinal lymph node
   D. CT chest, abdomen, pelvis

Viva Cases

Case 1

An 85-year-old man is referred to you for a recent diagnosis of squamous cell carcinoma of the penis. He had a preputial lesion that was excised completely by another urologist 3 weeks ago. On your exam, he has no additional lesions on the penis and has healed well from previous surgery. There were no palpable inguinal lymph nodes.

A. What are indications for inguinal lymph node dissection or sentinel lymph node biopsy in this patient?

Case 2

A 62-year-old man presents with a penile lesion and biopsy confirmed squamous cell carcinoma. On physical exam, you notice a 3 cm palpable, indurated, fixed lymph node in the right groin and a 2 cm mobile, indurated lymph node in the left groin.

A. What do you do next?

Case 3

A 75-year-old man present with a non-healing ulcer on the glans penis.

A. What are some risk factors for penile cancer?

Answers

Multiple Choice Questions

1. **C.** Men who have undergone neonatal circumcision are at lower risk of developing penile cancer.
2. **D.** SCC of the penis is associated with HPV 16 and 18 infections.

3. **B.** Extramammary Paget disease is an adenocarcinoma of the skin. It presents as a slowly expanding erythematous patch that is often pruritic. On pathology, it is characterized by Paget cells which are mucin positive and stain for low molecular weight cytokeratins (CK7 and CK20), GCDFP-15, periodic acid-Schiff (PAS) and carcinoembryonic antigen (CEA) [25].
4. **A.** Size of the primary lesion is not included in AJCC TNM staging.
5. **A.** Tumour invading into corpus spongiosum (either glans or ventral shaft) with or without urethral invasion is considered pT2. ≤2 unilateral inguinal metastases with no ENE is classified as pN1. Patient has no distant metastasis on imaging therefore he is M0.
6. **C.** This patient has high risk of occult inguinal lymph node metastasis. Invasive ILN staging is recommended.
7. **D.** This patient needs to undergo radiographic staging to rule out distant metastasis before proceeding with invasive staging and treatment.

Viva Cases

Case 1

A. Penile cancer follows a predictable pattern of drainage to the superficial inguinal lymph nodes followed by the deep inguinal lymph nodes. Staging inguinal lymph node dissection or sentinel lymph node biopsy should be performed to rule out microscopic metastasis in high-risk patient who have the following features in the primary tumor:
   - ≥ G2pT1 disease or
   - pT1 with lymphovascular invasion, perineural invasion, or high-grade histology (grade 3 or sarcomatoid)

Case 2

A. This patient needs additional staging work up to rule out distant metastasis. An abdominopelvic CT scan can be used to assess for pelvic and/or retroperitoneal lymphadenopathy as well as distant intra-abdominal metastasis. Thoracic CT should be obtained for additional chest staging. Alternative, PET/CT can be used to detect metastatic pelvic lymph nodes and/or distant metastasis in patients with advanced disease such has this patient with clinical evidence of inguinal lymph node metastasis. Ultrasound of the inguinal nodes_+/− fine needle aspiration of abnormal nodes is also required.

Case 3

A. Lack of neonatal circumcision with phimosis, chronic inflammation, lichen sclerosus, tobacco use, obesity, poor hygiene, exposure to UV radiation, history of sexually transmitted diseases, and human papillomavirus (HPV) infection, immunodeficiency.

Test your learning and check your understanding of this book's contents: use the "Springer Nature Flashcards" app to access questions using ▶ https://sn.pub/1r7Om8. To use the app, please follow the instructions in chapter 1.

References

1. Douglawi A, Masterson TA. Updates on the epidemiology and risk factors for penile cancer. Transl Androl Urol. 2017;6(5):785–90.
2. Hernandez BY, Barnholtz-Sloan J, German RR, Giuliano A, Goodman MT, King JB, et al. Burden of invasive squamous cell carcinoma of the penis in the United States, 1998-2003. Cancer. 2008;113(10 Suppl):2883–91.
3. Pow-Sang MR, Ferreira U, Pow-Sang JM, Nardi AC, Destefano V. Epidemiology and natural history of penile cancer. Urology. 2010;76(2 Suppl 1):S2–6.
4. Olesen TB, Sand FL, Rasmussen CL, Albieri V, Toft BG, Norrild B, et al. Prevalence of human papillomavirus DNA and p16(INK4a) in penile cancer and penile intraepithelial neoplasia: a systematic review and meta-analysis. Lancet Oncol. 2019;20(1):145–58.
5. Sufrin JR, Spiess AJ, Kramer DL, Libby PR, Miller JT, Bernacki RJ, et al. Targeting 5′-deoxy-5′-(methylthio)adenosine phosphorylase by 5′-haloalkyl analogues of 5′-deoxy-5′-(methylthio)adenosine. J Med Chem. 1991;34(8):2600–6.
6. Rishi A, Saini AS, Spiess PE, Yu A, Fernandez DC, Johnstone PAS, et al. Novel portable apparatus for outpatient high-dose-rate (HDR) brachytherapy in penile cancer. Brachytherapy. 2022;
7. Sanchez DF, Fernandez-Nestosa MJ, Canete-Portillo S, Rodriguez I, Cubilla AL. What is new in the pathologic staging of penile carcinoma in the 8th edition of AJCC TNM model: rationale for changes with practical stage-by-stage category diagnostic considerations. Adv Anat Pathol. 2021;28(4):209–27.
8. Horenblas S, Van Tinteren H, Delemarre JF, Moonen LM, Lustig V, Kroger R. Squamous cell carcinoma of the penis: accuracy of tumor, nodes and metastasis classification system, and role of lymphangiography, computerized tomography scan and fine needle aspiration cytology. J Urol. 1991;146(5):1279–83.
9. Cabanas RM. An approach for the treatment of penile carcinoma. Cancer. 1977;39(2):456–66.
10. Leijte JA, Kirrander P, Antonini N, Windahl T, Horenblas S. Recurrence patterns of squamous cell carcinoma of the penis: recommendations for follow-up based on a two-centre analysis of 700 patients. Eur Urol. 2008;54(1):161–8.
11. Lont AP, Kroon BK, Gallee MP, van Tinteren H, Moonen LM, Horenblas S. Pelvic lymph node dissection for penile carcinoma: extent of inguinal lymph node involvement as an indicator for pelvic lymph node involvement and survival. J Urol. 2007;177(3):947–52. discussion 52
12. Ravi R. Correlation between the extent of nodal involvement and survival following groin dissection for carcinoma of the penis. Br J Urol. 1993;72(5 Pt 2):817–9.
13. Hakenberg O, Comperat EM, Minhas S, Necchi A, Protzel C, Watkin N. EAU Guidelines on Penile Cancer. 2022.
14. National Comprehensive Cancer Network. Penile cancer (Version 2.2020). Retrieved from https://www.nccn.org/professionals/physician_gls/pdf/penile.pdf.
15. Graafland NM, Lam W, Leijte JA, Yap T, Gallee MP, Corbishley C, et al. Prognostic factors for occult inguinal lymph node involvement in penile carcinoma and assessment of the high-risk EAU subgroup: a two-institution analysis of 342 clinically node-negative patients. Eur Urol. 2010;58(5):742–7.
16. Ottenhof SR, Vegt E. The role of PET/CT imaging in penile cancer. Transl Androl Urol. 2017;6(5):833–8.

17. Fletcher JW, Djulbegovic B, Soares HP, Siegel BA, Lowe VJ, Lyman GH, et al. Recommendations on the use of 18F-FDG PET in oncology. J Nucl Med. 2008;49(3):480–508.
18. Scher B, Seitz M, Reiser M, Hungerhuber E, Hahn K, Tiling R, et al. 18F-FDG PET/CT for staging of penile cancer. J Nucl Med. 2005;46(9):1460–5.
19. Leijte JA, Graafland NM, Valdes Olmos RA, van Boven HH, Hoefnagel CA, Horenblas S. Prospective evaluation of hybrid 18F-fluorodeoxyglucose positron emission tomography/computed tomography in staging clinically node-negative patients with penile carcinoma. BJU Int. 2009;104(5):640–4.
20. Souillac I, Rigaud J, Ansquer C, Marconnet L, Bouchot O. Prospective evaluation of (18) F-fluorodeoxyglucose positron emission tomography-computerized tomography to assess inguinal lymph node status in invasive squamous cell carcinoma of the penis. J Urol. 2012;187(2):493–7.
21. Sadeghi R, Gholami H, Zakavi SR, Kakhki VR, Horenblas S. Accuracy of 18F-FDG PET/CT for diagnosing inguinal lymph node involvement in penile squamous cell carcinoma: systematic review and meta-analysis of the literature. Clin Nucl Med. 2012;37(5):436–41.
22. Krishna RP, Sistla SC, Smile R, Krishnan R. Sonography: an underutilized diagnostic tool in the assessment of metastatic groin nodes. J Clin Ultrasound. 2008;36(4):212–7.
23. Culkin DJ, Beer TM. Advanced penile carcinoma. J Urol. 2003;170(2 Pt 1):359–65.
24. Lughezzani G, Catanzaro M, Torelli T, Piva L, Biasoni D, Stagni S, et al. The relationship between characteristics of inguinal lymph nodes and pelvic lymph node involvement in penile squamous cell carcinoma: a single institution experience. J Urol. 2014;191(4):977–82.
25. St Claire K, Hoover A, Ashack K, Khachemoune A. Extramammary Paget disease. Dermatol Online J. 2019;25:4.

5 Premalignant Penile Lesions

Thomas T. F. Wong, Martin Mak, Hussain M Alnajjar, and Wayne Lam

Learning Objectives

After reading this chapter you will be able to:

- Outline risk factors for the development of premalignant penile lesions
- Define common human papillomavirus-related and non-human papillomavirus-related premalignant penile lesions
- Describe the natural history of some premalignant penile lesions
- Discuss both non-invasive and invasive treatment options for premalignant penile lesions

T. T. F. Wong · M. Mak
Division of Urology, Department of Surgery, Queen Mary Hospital, Pokfulam, Hong Kong SAR

H. M Alnajjar
Department of Urology, Institute of Andrology, University College London Hospital, London, UK

W. Lam (✉)
Division of Urology, Department of Surgery, Queen Mary Hospital, Pokfulam, Hong Kong SAR

Division of Urology, Department of Surgery, LKS Faculty of Medicine, The University of Hong Kong, Pokfulam, Hong Kong SAR
e-mail: lamwayne@hku.hk

O. Brunckhorst et al. (eds.), *Penile Cancer – A Practical Guide*, Management of Urology, https://doi.org/10.1007/978-3-031-32681-3_5

Table 5.1 Examples of HPV related and non-HPV related premailignant penile lesions

HPV related	Penile intraepithelial neoplasia Giant Condyloma Acuminatum (Buschke-Löwenstein tumour)
Non-HPV related	Lichen sclerosus (Balanitis Xerotica Obliterans) Pseudoepitheliomatous Keratotic and Micaceous Balanitis Cutaneous horn

Introduction

Premalignant penile lesions are often a diagnostic challenge. They account for up to 10% of all penile malignancies at first presentation [1]. Many of which are difficult to distinguish from benign penile dermatological diseases. Patient presentations are often delayed, likely due to lack of awareness, fear, and patient embarrassment. Not uncommonly, patients have a history of unsuccessful self-management. Subsequently, delayed presentation and treatment may result in disease progression to invasive carcinoma reported in up to 33% if left untreated [2].

The rarity of this disease has made data acquisition for research limited. Standardisation of clinical practice has, therefore, been challenging. The natural history of many premalignant penile lesions remains uncertain. Malignant transformation into invasive carcinoma may result in patients requiring more aggressive and extensive treatment [3]. To prevent this, early recognition and prompt treatment have been acknowledged as the best approach to the management of premalignant penile lesions.

Several risk factors have been recognized to be associated with the development and progression of premalignant penile lesion. These include the presence of a foreskin, poor hygiene, phimosis, smoking, chronic inflammation, lichen sclerosus and in men with multiple sexual partners.

Premalignant penile lesions can broadly be classified as Human Papilloma Virus (HPV) related which is the most important risk factor most widely investigated, and those that are non-HPV related commonly due to chronic inflammation (Table 5.1).

Human Papillomavirus-Related Lesions

Penile Intraepithelial Neoplasia

Carcinoma in situ (CIS) of penis is also known as penile intraepithelial neoplasia (PeIN) (Fig. 5.1). Erythroplasia of Queyrat (EQ) is PeIN lesion that involves the glans penis and inner prepuce, whereas Bowen's disease (BD) is reserved for penile shaft lesions. Bowenoid papulosis (BP) is the third entity described by Kopf and Bart, and it is a condition having a similar histologic appearance to PeIN but runs a benign course. The three lesions fall into the category of penile intraepithelial neoplasia but have distinct clinical features and characteristics [4]. There is strong link between human papillomavirus infection and undifferentiated PeIN [5].

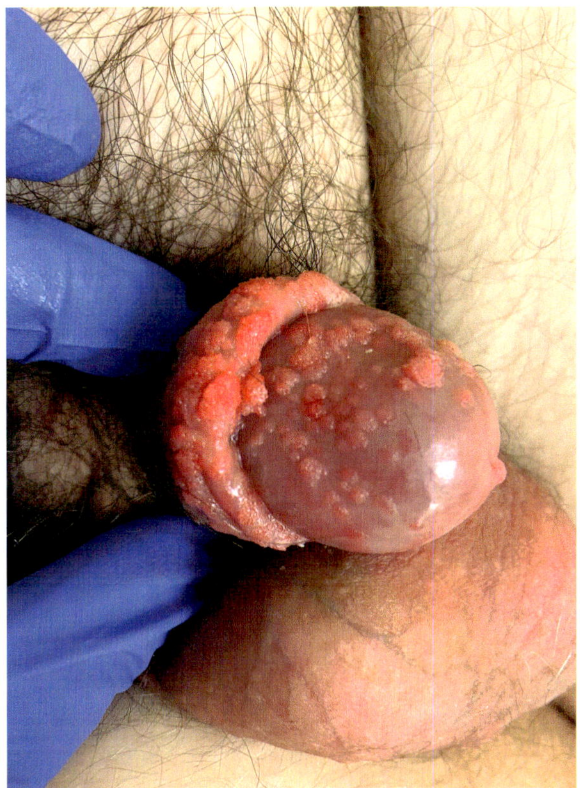

Fig. 5.1 Penile intraepithelial neoplasia (PeIN) of the glans and inner foreskin

BP usually affects patients in the third or fourth decade of life. It manifests as multiple papules with a pigmented surface [6]. It is frequently misdiagnosed as condyloma accuminatum, and biopsy is warranted to confirm the diagnosis. Histologically this condition is a PeIN, but it rarely progresses to invasive cancer and is generally considered not precancerous. Unlike condyloma accuminatum which is associated with HPV-6 and 11, this lesion commonly contains high risk subtypes such as HPV-16 or 18 [7]. Treatment includes excision, cryotherapy, laser fulguration and topical 5-fluorouracil/Imiquimod creams.

EQ typically manifests as an erythematous, well-marginated lesion on the glans penis or inner prepuce of uncircumcised men. It is a rare condition and usually occurs in the fourth and fifth decade of life, with an average age of 49 [8]. The lesion can ulcerate and be associated with pain and discharge [9]. BD is characterised by sharply defined plaques of scaly erythema on the penile shaft. Progression into invasive penile cancer is more common in EQ ~30% [9] compared to BD ~5% [2].

Interestingly, in countries with a low incidence of penile cancer, PeIN predominates over invasive lesions, whereas in countries with a high incidence of penile cancer, PeIN is usually associated with invasive cancer. Like in invasive penile cancer, PeIN can be classified from a pathogenic point of view into HPV-related and non-HPV-related. The former group includes undifferentiated subtypes namely basaloid, warty and warty-basaloid, while the latter group encompasses usual, verrucous, papillary, sarcomatoid, pseudohyperplastic, and cuniculatum carcinomas [10]. Another difference is that more than half of the patients with differentiated PeIN have a history of lichen sclerosus. Basaloid or warty subtypes are rarely associated with lichen sclerosus.

The prevalence of HPV infection in PeIN is between 87–100% of cases, which is more common than in penile cancer [11]. Other risk factors for PeIN include inflammatory skin disease (OR 14.7, 95% CI 6.5–33.4), diseases of the prepuce (OR 4.0, 95% CI 2.2–7.4), immunosuppressive drugs (OR 5.0, 95% CI 2.5–9.8), penile surgical procedures (OR 4.8, 95% CI 2.2–10.8), balanitis (OR 9.2, 95% CI 5.0–16.8), genital warts (9.9, 95% CI 4.3–22.7) and organ transplantation (7.0, 95% CI 2.4–20.8) [12]. Poor socio-economical status, or single men, have been suggested as risk factors for penile cancer, but not for PeIN [12].

Giant Condyloma Acuminatum (Buschke-Löwenstein Tumour)

Buschke-Löwenstein tumour (BLT) is different from Condyloma acuminatum in that the latter always remains superficial and does not invade adjacent tissues. Giant condyloma usually presents with a large and slow-growing exophytic cauliflower-like lesion that can at times become extensive, leading to the invasion and formation fistula with the urethra and rectum in extreme cases. The histopathology typically gives a benign appearance resembling condyloma acuminatum, but BLT can be recognised by its thicker stratum corneum, the marked papillary proliferations, and its tendency to invade deeply, displacing the underlying tissues. These same features are seen in verrucous carcinoma and some authors do not recognize a distinction between it and BLTs [13]. As with condyloma acuminata, DNA from HPV 6 and 11 has been recovered from the BLT [14]. In the review published by Chu et al. [15], perianal tumour has a significant association with existing carcinoma (56%) and a high recurrence rate (67%). The mainstay of treatment is radical surgical excision with wide margins. Skin graft reconstruction may be necessary in extensive cases.

HPV Infection and Malignant Transformation

Studies have shown a prevalence of 20% or higher in anogenital samples of men [16]. Most HPV infections remain asymptomatic, and up to 70% are cleared within 1 year. Unlike in females where HPV infection appears to cause all cervical cancer, HPV infection only causes a portion of penile cancer in men. HPV 6,11 and 42 to 44 are low risk types and associated with condylomata and low-grade dysplasia. HPV 16, 18, 31, 33, 35, 39, 45, 51, 52, 58 and 59 are high risk types with 16 being by far the commonest to be associated with malignant disease [17].

HPV viruses are oncogenic because of the viral proteins E6 and E7. Data suggests that E6 and E7 bind to tumour suppressor gene products TP53 and pRB (retinoblastoma protein). The inhibitory effect on TP53 leads to chromosome instability,

DNA mutations and aneuploidy, whereas the activity on pRB causes upregulation of $p16^{Ink4a}$, which drives cell cycle progression. Stankiewicz [18] showed that the pRB – $p16^{Ink4a}$ pathway but not the p53 is disrupted by HPV infection in penile cancer. The strong positive correlation between $p16^{Ink4a}$ and HPV detection has led to the use of $p16^{Ink4a}$ in immunostaining as a mean of HPV testing. Meta-analysis showed that $p16^{INK4a}$ is positive in 49.5% cases of PeIN [19].

In one RCT, the efficacy of quadrivalent HPV vaccine against genital lesions related to HPV-6, 11, 16 or 18 was 90.4% in per-protocol population [20]. No PeIN developed in the vaccination arm. Although circumcision is a known protective factor against penile cancer, the evidence whether it lowers the incidence of HPV infection is unclear. A large multinational study showed no significant difference in incidence and clearance of HPV infection in circumscribed men [21].

Non-Human Papillomavirus-Related Lesions

Lichen Sclerosus (Balanitis Xerotica Obliterans)

Lichen sclerosus (LSc) et atrophicus a chronic inflammatory mucocutaneous disease with unknown etiology. The lesion manifests as a whitish patch on the prepuce of glans, sometimes extending to the meatus and fossa navicularis, or even severe urethral stricture disease in extreme cases. It can cause pruritus, pain, dyspareunia and bleeding. In severe cases, it can cause phimosis and stricture of the urethra. One study demonstrated 58.7% incidence of lichen sclerosus observed in histopathology diagnosis from 351 patients undergoing circumcision for symptomatic preputium [22]. A recent study demonstrated that accentuated contact between urine and susceptible penile epithelium due to occlusion can lead to male genital lichen sclerosus [23].

In most of the cases, a clinical diagnosis can be made with the symptoms and signs of lichen sclerosus. The most significant risk factor is the lack of circumcision. A study showed that the age-adjusted odds ratio of 53.55 (95% confidence interval [CI]: 7.24–395.88) for uncircumcised males to have LSc [24]. Injuries to the foreskin such as trauma, piercing and previous surgeries also lead to significant increased risk of LSc. Another case series has further strengthened the urinary occlusion hypothesis for the causation of male genital lichen sclerosus. The study concluded that urological interventions can create incompetence of the naviculomeatal valve post voiding and in uncircumcised men, this creates a risk factor for LSc [25].

The risk of malignant transformation into SCC of the penis is approximately 4–8% [26]. There are reports that describe the development of SCC penis years after treatment for LSc [27, 28]. LSc is also a common concomitant finding in penile cancer pathology, in 28–50% of cases [29, 30].

A number of studies have investigated the genetic basis of LSc and the predominant evaluation is on the human leukocyte antigen (HLA) genotypes [31]. The most common association is HLA-DQ7, but overall, these studies did not identify a specific genetic profile that predisposes to the disease.

The three competing theories for the development of LSc are infective, autoimmune and chronic irritations [29]. Infectious microorganisms that have been investigated or identified include Borrelia burgdorferi, Epstein Barr Virus, Human Papilloma Virus and hepatitis C virus. So far, there is not enough evidence to suggest that either of them is a causative agent to the development in LSc.

Some clinicians may consider a trial of topical corticosteroids in milder cases, although its efficacy especially in the adult population is generally poor. Topical Clobetasol propionate 0.05% ointment should be given once per day for 1 month [32, 33]. Circumcision, whereby microenvironment causing irritations is eliminated, have been reported to provide a good long-term cure rate [34]. In patients with persistent or severe glans penis involvement despite circumcision, surgery with glans-resurfacing and split-thickness skin grafting should be considered. In more severe cases with associated urethral stricture, urethral reconstructive surgery, often with the use of buccal mucosa graft, or perineal urethrostomy, should be considered.

Pseudoepitheliomatous Keratotic and Micaceous Balanitis

Pseudoepitheliomatous Keratotic and Micaceous Balanitis is a rare condition that presents as a single, well-demarcated, hyperkeratotic micaceous growth on the surface of the glans penis in older men [35]. Patients may complain of difficulty retracting the prepuce. The exact etiology for this lesion is not fully understood.

It is characterized histologically by acanthosis, hyperkeratosis and pseudoepitheliomatous hyperplasia. PEKMB represents a form of chronic, undiagnosed or misdiagnosed, inadequately treated or treatment refractory, unstable lichen sclerosus. The significant potential for squamous carcinogenesis (differentiated PeIN and verrucous carcinoma) can be mitigated by timely diagnosis and treatment. Glans resurfacing and split skin graft reconstruction appears to be a successful treatment modality in patients with refractory disease [36].

Cutaneous Horn

Cutaneous horn is a dermatological condition in which a keratinized protrusion is developed above the skin, mostly at the face or scalp. Cutaneous horn of the penis has been described but limited to case reports due to its rarity. Cutaneous horn usually presents as a solid protuberance on the glans, characterized by cornification of the epithelium. It typically develops from a pre-existing skin lesion. Predisposing factors include trauma, infection, chronic inflammation, and previous surgeries. It is important to obtain the histology of the base of the cutaneous horn, as this may have an impact on further management. A study reported that penile horn might be benign in 42–56% of cases, premalignant in 22–37% or malignant in 20–22% [37]. The mainstay of treatment is complete surgical excision.

Treatment of Premalignant Penile Lesions

Topical Therapies—5-Fluorouracil

5% 5-fluorouracil (5-FU) is an antimetabolite chemotherapeutic pyrimidine analogue that act by inhibiting thymidylate synthase with resultant DNA damage [38]. It is reported to be one of the most used first line treatments. Earlier studies of 5-FU showed promising results with 100% complete response and no recurrence up to 70 months of follow-up [39, 40]. A more recent study that included 42 PeIN patients treated with topical 5-FU showed complete response rate of 50% over a mean follow-up of 34 months and recurrence rate of 20% with a mean time to recurrence of 5 months [41]. Progression after 5-FU was reported to be 11% [42]. There is no standardised regimen for application, but typically the cream is applied to the lesion for 12 h every 48 h for 4–6 weeks. Side effects appear to be tolerable and include pain, irritation, redness, and hypersensitivity [43].

Topical Therapies—Imiquimod

Imiquimod is an immunomodulating drug that activates macrophages and other cells to stimulate both innate and cell mediated immune systems mainly via Toll-like receptor 7 agonism. This ultimately results in immune defense against both viral infected cells and tumor cells [44]. A review included 48 patients with PeIN treated with imiquimod showed an overall complete response of 63%, partial response in 8% and no response in 29% and recurrence rate of 4% with a mean follow-up of 12 months. Complete response rate varied between different PeIN clinical subtypes; penile Bowen's disease (88%), Bowenoid papulosis (75%) and erythroplasia of Queyrat (53%). Progression after imiquimod was reported to be 20% [42]. Furthermore, regimes of fewer than four applications per week over 3–4 months had a higher complete response rate at 81% compared to patients who had more than four applications per week over 1–2 months with a complete response of 68%. Adverse events include erythema, vesiculation, scrotal ulceration, bleeding, headache, flu like symptoms and myalgia [45].

Cryotherapy

Cryotherapy with liquid nitrogen utilises rapid freeze/slow thaw cycles to achieve temperatures between -20C and -50C to cause tissue damage by ice crystals formation, leading to disruption of cell membranes and cell death [46]. A study of 299 patients with extragenital BD found a greater risk of recurrence after cryotherapy (13.4%) compared with 5-FU (9%) and surgical excision (5.5%) following 5 years of follow-up [47]. In an attempt to improve the outcome of cryotherapy, Shaw et al. hypothesized the synergistic effect of combining cryotherapy and topical imiquimod. They reported a case series of 8 PeIN patients and all had complete response with no recurrence at mean follow-up of 25 months. However, the excellent outcome might be attributed by concurrent treatment with topical 5-FU or laser therapies in 4 out of 8 patients [48].

Laser Therapy

Laser treatments are an attractive penile preserving therapy compared to topical therapy as it does not rely on patient's compliance, which is pivotal for a chance of complete response. Although it is associated with minimal morbidity and better cosmetic outcome than surgery, it had variable results with recurrence rate ranging from 10–48.3%. This is potentially due to the lesion being under-staged due to under-sampling at initial biopsy for diagnosis.

A commonly used medium, CO_2, allows precise vaporisation of affected areas with depth of penetration up to 2–2.5 mm. The lower depth of destruction results in better preservation of tissue for histological examination. Conversely, this can also result in inadequate ablation of lesions in one session and subsequent recurrence. A study which included 106 patients with pTis disease, evaluating peniscopically controlled CO2 therapy, demonstrated a cumulative risk of recurrence at 5 years of 10%, with a secondary partial penectomy rate of 3% [49]. Another study of 58 PeIN patients treated with lasers had recurrence in 48.3% with median follow-up of 63.8 months [50].

Alternatively, Nd:YAG laser penetrates the skin to cause coagulation at a depth of 3–10 mm, it usually cannot be used to provide tissue for histological diagnosis due to its coagulation effect. Studies on Nd:YAG laser treatment with follow-up of more than 3 years reported variable local recurrence rates ranging from 10 to 48% [51–53]. The rate of secondary partial penectomy after initial treatment was reported at 45% in one series [51].

The most common side effects following laser therapy for premalignant penile lesions include pain during the administration of the therapy, or meatal stenosis in perimeatal lesions. Complete re-epithelialization would be expected in 2–4 weeks with reported excellent cosmetic outcomes [50].

Photodynamic Therapy

Photodynamic therapy (PDT) involves application of a topical photosensitising cream containing chemicals such as delta-5-aminolevulinic acid (ALA) or methyl aminolevulinate (MAL) to affected area, followed by illumination with light from an incoherent source, leading to photo selective cell death of sensitised cells. Recent review of 69 PeIN patients treated with PDT, it demonstrated varied results with complete response ranging from 47.6–62.5%. Cosmetic preservation appeared excellent with PDT. PDT is not commonly utilized in modern clinical practice. Commonly reported adverse effects included temporary tingling, burning, pain, or other discomfort during and after the therapy [54].

Surgical Excision

Surgical treatment of premalignant penile lesions remains the mainstay treatment of choice. It is especially suitable in patients who have extensive disease involvement, those with recurrent disease following topical or conservative treatments, and in patients who may be difficult to be compliant with topical treatment or surveillance post-treatment. Surgical excision also allows the lesion to be thoroughly examined histologically to ensure no focus of invasive malignancy has been under-sampled during the initial incisional biopsy. To help delineate margins of penile lesions and to help visualize occult lesions intra-operatively, some clinicians advocate the application of topical 5% acetic acid for 5-minutes to achieve the 'aceto-white' reactions.

For patients with premalignant penile lesions confined to the prepuce, it serves to excise the lesions that are confined to the prepuce by circumcision. This also fundamentally eliminates the micro-environment that harbors chronic HPV infection and chronic inflammation, both of which may contribute to the progression of disease into invasive malignancy over time.

Historically, Moh's micrographic surgery (MMS) has been used for many common skin cancers since 1930s, and it has been adopted to treat patients with premalignant penile lesions [55]. MMS has also been used to excise penile lesions. The procedure involves the use of microscopic excision of the lesion in thin horizontal layers. Concurrent multiple frozen sections are taken for microscopic evaluation until resection margins are deemed clear. This technique allows maximal organ preservation giving excellence cosmetic and functional outcomes, but is often very time consuming, requiring dedicated trained collaborative surgeons and pathologists to achieve oncological clearance. The reported recurrence rate is high at 32% [56], and the use of MMS in treatment of men with penile lesions has been limited.

For patients with significant disease involving the glans penis, a partial or total glans resurfacing procedure has gained popularity (Fig. 5.2). Glans resurfacing was first described by Bracka for the treatment of extensive balanitis xerotica obliterans (BXO) [57]. Its use has since been adopted not only in the management of other premalignant penile lesions, but also both patients with glandular PeIN and invasive tumours of up to stage T1a disease [58–61]. Glans resurfacing provides optimal preservation of penile length, with good functional and cosmetic outcomes.

The procedure is typically carried out under a general anaesthesia with a penile block, or under spinal anaesthesia. A penile tourniquet is then applied. All epithelium and sub-epithelium of the glans are excised from the spongiosum using sharp dissection in quadrants, starting from the meatus towards the coronal sulcus. In selected patients, corpus spongiosum deep biopsies are taken for frozen section to confirm margin clearance or if invasive disease is suspected intra-operatively. The distal margin of the remaining prepuce is secured to the sub-coronal level of the shaft penis with interrupted 4/0 vicryl rapide. The excised specimen is often fragile and should be handled with care, cautiously mounted on a foam or film oriented to guide pathologists for accurate pathological assessment. (Fig. 5.3).

A split thickness skin graft (STSG) is then harvested, usually from the thigh, using an air dermatome. The graft is trimmed and is sutured on to the skin edges,

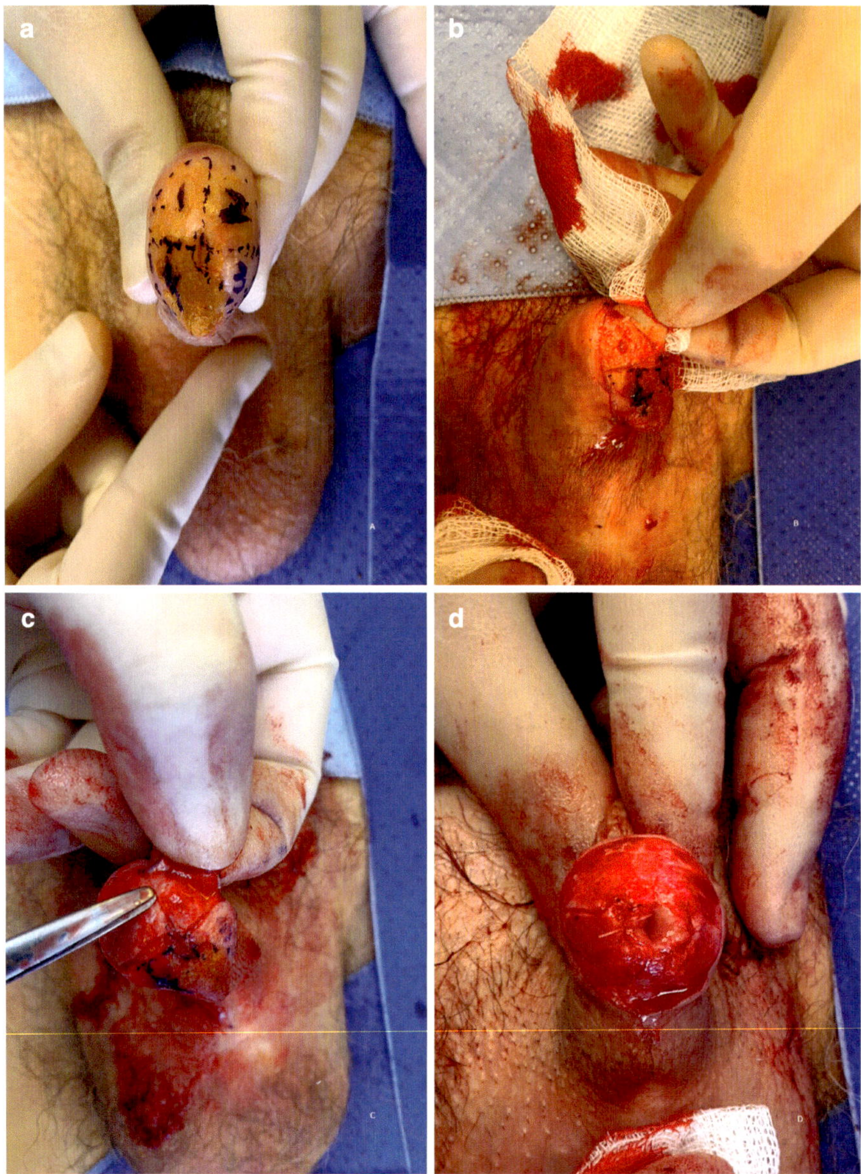

Fig. 5.2 Total glans resurfacing for a patient with PeIN. (**a**) 4 quadrants marker done with the meatus marked separately; (**b**, **c**): Individual quadrants are excised carefully by dissecting the epithelial and subepithelial layers (**d**) The denuded glans with a spatulated neomeatus

covering the denuded glans, using interrupted 4/0 and 5/0 vicryl rapde sutures (Fig. 5.4). Quilting sutures with 5/0 vicryle rapide are also applied to ensure graft adherence. A 14 Ch urethral catheter is inserted to divert urine away from the surgical site to keep the wound dry and clean post-operatively. A TODGA dressing is

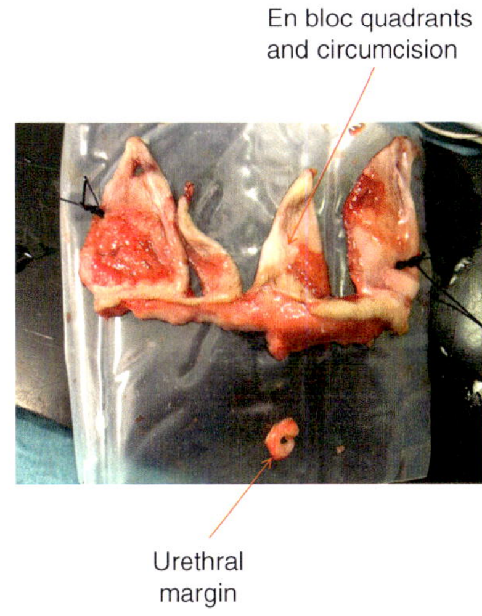

Fig. 5.3 Mounting of specimen mounted on a plastic surface to assist with more accurate pathological assessment. A separate meatal margin was also taken

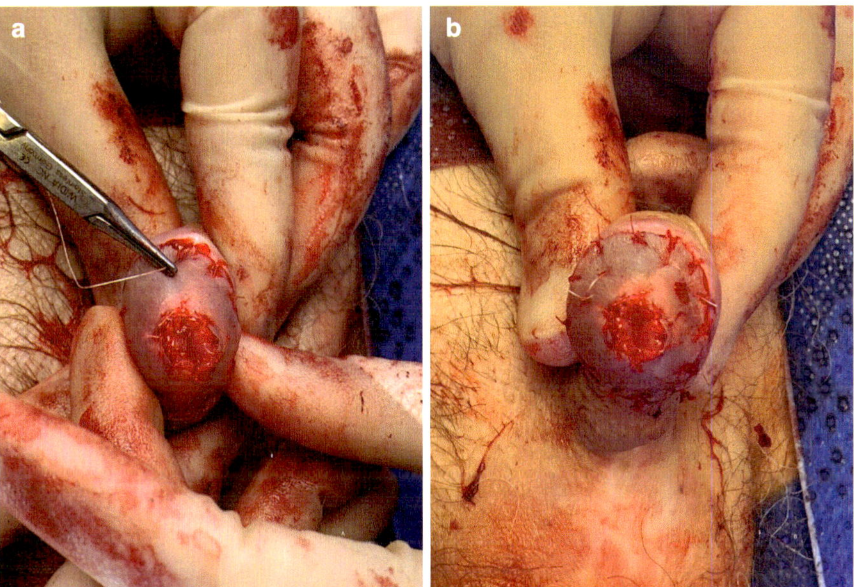

Fig. 5.4 Split thickness graft post excision. (**a**) Split thickness graft is applied onto the denuded spongy tissue of the glans; (**b**) The neoglans with a split thickness skin graft and quilted sutures to allow graft take

applied to the neoglans to secure the graft and allow graft take. Both dressings and catheter are removed on post-op day 10 [62].

Partial glans resurfacing and coronal sparing glans resurfacing could be considered in patients with isolated foci of penile premalignant lesion with less than 50% of glans involvement or where the corona is not involved, maximising glans sensation and cosmesis. The surgical principle of partial glans resurfacing is similar to that of total glans resurfacing. A wedge of glans epithelium and its underlying sub-epithelium excised from the spongiosum prior to the application of a STSG. This approach also aims to preserve a degree of normal glans skin and associated sensation [63].

The advantage of glans resurfacing is that it is able to provide both diagnostic and therapeutic abilities. It enables accurate histopathological staging, excluding disease being more advanced than anticipated. In a study of 25 patients with PeIN treated with total glans resurfacing, 40% of patient were found to have invasive cancer on final pathological analysis, different from the initial incisional biopsy findings [59]. 4% were found to have local recurrence at a mean follow up of 29 months. In another small series of 10 patients with glans PeIN, none of the patients were found to have disease recurrence after a mean follow up of 30 months [58].

Follow up

Currently, there is no standardized follow-up protocols recommended in any guidelines following treatment of this rare condition. It should be highly dependent on the type of premalignant lesion and treatment used. However, cautious, tailored follow-up should be arranged for these patients, together with robust patient education with regular self-examinations, given the uncertain natural history of most of the described premalignant lesions and the associated 33% reported malignant transformation rate. The authors recommend patients should be followed up in clinic every 3 months for the initial year, 4 monthly for the second year after treatment, then 6 monthly for up to at least 5 years post-treatment.

Key Points

- Premalignant penile lesions can broadly be classified as Human Papilloma Virus (HPV) related and non-HPV related
- There is strong link between human papillomavirus infection and penile intraepithelial neoplasia.
- The three competing theories for the development of Lichen sclerosus are infective, autoimmune, and chronic irritations.
- Treatment of premalignant penile lesions generally include topical therapies, cryotherapy, laser, photodynamic therapy, and surgical excision.
- Surgical treatment, most commonly by glans resurfacing with partial thickness skin graft, remains the mainstay treatment of choice for premalignant lesions, especially for patients with extensive disease involvement, failed topical treatment or poor compliance with surveillance

Revisions Questions

Multiple Choice Questions

1. Which of the following premalignant penile lesions is HPV-related?
   A. Lichen sclerosus
   B. Pseudoepitheliomatous keratotic and micaceous balanitis
   C. Buschke-Löwenstein Tumour
   D. Cutaneous horn
2. Which of the following lesions is the least likely to progress into penile cancer?
   A. Bowenoid papulosis
   B. Lichen sclerosus
   C. Buschke-Löwenstein Tumour
   D. Cutaneous horn
3. Which of the following should be the most preferred surgical treatment for erythroplasia of Queyrat involving the glans penis?
   A. Total penectomy
   B. Partial penectomy
   C. Glansectomy
   D. Glans-resurfacing with partial thickness skin graft
4. Which of the following best describes Buschke-Löwenstein Tumour?
   A. It does not invade adjacent tissues
   B. Topical treatment is often the first-line treatment
   C. The histology may resemble that of condyloma acuminatum
   D. It manifests as a whitish patch on the prepuce

Viva Case

Case 1

A 50-year-old gentleman presents with a 2 years history of whitish lesion on the glans penis and complains of lower urinary tract symptoms.

A. How would you assess this patient?
B. What would you offer to treat his condition?
C. What is Koebner phenomenon? What is the significance of this if we are to treat this patient with surgery?

Answers

Multiple Choice Questions

1. **C.** Buschke-Löwenstein Tumour, also known as giant condyloma acuminatum, is associated with HPV virus most commonly type 6 and 11.

2. **A**. Bowenoid papulosis has a similar histologic appearance to carcinoma in-situ but it runs a benign course.
3. **D**. Glans resurfacing with partial thickness skin graft should be offered If possible because it preserves the optimal penile length, with good functional and cosmetic outcomes.
4. **C**. Buschke-Löwenstein Tumour often manifests as a large or extensive lesion that can invade into adjacent tissues. The histology may resemble condyloma acuminatum, but BLT can be recognised by its thicker stratum corneum, the marked papillary proliferations, and its tendency to invade deeply, displacing the underlying tissues.

Viva Case

Case 1

It is a patient with lichen sclerosus.

A. I would enquire about the onset and duration of the lesion, whether it is enlarging and associated with any pain or bleeding. I will ask specifically about voiding symptoms and hematuria. I will ask specifically for risks factors including phimosis, balanitis, trauma to the penis, piercing or previous surgery. In physical examination, I will assess the relation of the lesion to prepuce, corpus, and urethra. I will measure the stretched penile length. If there is suspicion of co-existing penile cancer, I will also palpate for any inguinal lymph nodes. I will perform an abdominal exam to rule out organomegaly and palpate for any supraclavicular lymph nodes. For investigations, I will perform a uroflowmetry and urethroscopy to assess for any stricture.

B. Treatment is by topical steroids or surgery. Some clinicians offer topical Clobetasol propionate 0.05% ointment given once per day for 1–3 months. Surgical treatment include circumcision +/− glans resurfacing with partial thickness skin graft. Urethral stricturing disease may require reconstructive surgery.

C. The Koebner phenomenon describes appearance of skin lesions on the lines of trauma. It is important to avoid using penile skin graft when we operate for lichen sclerosus.

Test your learning and check your understanding of this book's contents: use the "Springer Nature Flashcards" app to access questions using ▶ https://sn.pub/1r7Om8. To use the app, please follow the instructions in chapter 1.

References

1. Brown CT, Minhas S, Ralph DJ. Conservative surgery for penile cancer: subtotal glans excision without grafting. BJU Int. 2005;96(6):911–2.
2. Wieland U, Jurk S, Weissenborn S, Krieg T, Pfister H, Ritzkowsky A. Erythroplasia of queyrat: coinfection with cutaneous carcinogenic human papillomavirus type 8 and genital papillomaviruses in a carcinoma in situ. J Invest Dermatol. 2000;115(3):396–401.
3. Dräger DL, Milerski S, Sievert KD, Hakenberg OW. Psychosoziale Auswirkungen bei Patienten mit Peniskarzinom: Ein systematischer Überblick [Psychosocial effects in patients with penile cancer : a systematic review]. Urologe A. 2018;57(4):444–52.
4. Porter WM, Francis N, Hawkins D, Dinneen M, Bunker CB. Penile intraepithelial neoplasia: clinical spectrum and treatment of 35 cases. Br J Dermatol. 2002;147(6):1159–65.
5. Canete-Portillo S, Sanchez DF, Cubilla AL. Pathology of invasive and intraepithelial penile neoplasia. Eur Urol Focus. 2019;5(5):713–7.
6. Patterson JW, Kao GF, Graham JH, Helwig EB. Bowenoid papulosis. A clinicopathologic study with ultrastructural observations. Cancer. 1986;57(4):823–36.
7. Schwartz RA, Janniger CK. Bowenoid papulosis. J Am Acad Dermatol. 1991;24:261.
8. Graham JH, Helwig EB. Erythroplasia of Queyrat: a clinicopathologic and histochemical study. Cancer. 1973;32:1396–414.
9. Goette DK. Review of erythroplasia of Queyrat and its treatment. Urology. 1976;8(4):311–5.
10. Velazquez EF, Chaux A, Cubilla AL. Histologic classification of penile intraepithelial neoplasia. Semin Diagn Pathol. 2012;29(2):96–102.
11. Kristiansen S, Svensson A, Drevin L, Forslund O, Torbrand C, Bjartling C. Risk factors for penile intraepithelial neoplasia: a population-based register study in Sweden, 2000-2012. Acta Derm Venereol. 2019;99(3):315–20.
12. Torbrand C, Wigertz A, Drevin L, Folkvaljon Y, Lambe M, Hakansson U, et al. Socioeconomic factors and penile cancer risk and mortality; a population-based study. BJU Int. 2017;119:254–60.
13. Bogomoletz WV, Potet F, Molas G. Condyloma acuminata, giant condyloma acuminatum (Buschke- Loewenstein tumour) and verrucous squamous carcinoma of the perianal and anorectal region: a continuous precancerous spectrum? Histopathology. 1985;9:1155–69.
14. Braga JC, Nadal SR, Stiepcich M, Framil VM, Muller H. Buschke-Loewenstein tumour: identification of HPV type 6 and 11. An Bras Dermatol. 2012;87(1):131–4.
15. Chu QD, Vezeridis MP, Libbey NP, et al. Giant condyloma acuminatum (Buschke-Lowenstein tumour) of the anorectal and perianal regions. Dis Colon Rectum. 1994;37:950–7.
16. Dunne EF, Nielson CM, Stone KM, Markowitz LE, Giuliano AR. Prevalence of HPV infection among men: a systematic review of the literature. J Infect Dis. 2006;194(8):1044–57.
17. Stratton KL, Culkin DJ. A contemporary review of HPV and penile cancer. Oncology. 2016;30(3):245–9
18. Stankiewicz E, Prowse DM, Ktori E, Cuzick J, Ambroisine L, Zhang X, Kudahetti S, Watkin N, Corbishley C, Berney DM. The retinoblastoma protein/p16 INK4A pathway but not p53 is disrupted by human papillomavirus in penile squamous cell carcinoma. Histopathology. 2011;58(3):433–9.
19. Olesen TB, Sand FL, Rasmussen CL, Albieri V, Toft BG, Norrild B, Munk C, Kjær SK. Prevalence of human papillomavirus DNA and p16INK4a in penile cancer and penile intraepithelial neoplasia: a systematic review and meta-analysis. Lancet Oncol. 2019;20(1):145–58.
20. Giuliano AR, Palefsky JM, Goldstone S, Moreira ED Jr, et al. Efficacy of quadrivalent HPV vaccine against HPV infection and disease in males. N Engl J Med. 2011;364(5):401–11.

21. Albero G, Castellsague X, Lin HY, et al. Male circumcision and the incidence and clearance of genital human papillomavirus (HPV) infection in men: the HPV infection in men (HIM) cohort study. BMC Infect Dis. 2014;14:75.
22. Kristiansen S, Bjartling C, Svensson Å, Forslund O, Torbrand C. Penile intraepithelial neoplasia, penile cancer precursors and human papillomavirus prevalence in symptomatic preputium: a cross-sectional study of 351 circumcised men in Sweden. BJU Int. 2021;127(4):428–34.
23. Kravvas G, Muneer A, Watchorn RE, Castiglione F, Haider A, Freeman A, Hadway P, Alnajjar H, Lynch M, Bunker CB. Male genital lichen sclerosus, microincontinence and occlusion: mapping the disease across the prepuce. Clin Exp Dermatol. 2022;47(6):1124–30.
24. Mallon E, Hawkins D, Dinneen M, et al. Circumcision and genital dermatoses. Arch Dermatol. 2000;136(3):350–4.
25. Panou E, Panagou E, Foley C, Kravvas G, Watchorn R, Alnajjar H, Muneer A, Bunker CB. Male genital lichen sclerosus associated with urological interventions and microincontinence: a case series of 21 patients. Clin Exp Dermatol. 2022;47(1):107–9.
26. Clouston D, Hall A, Lawrentschuk N. Penile lichen sclerosus (balanitis xerotica obliterans). BJU Int. 2011;108(Suppl 2):14–9.
27. Nasca MR, Innocenzi D, Micali G. Penile cancer among patients with genital lichen sclerosus. J Am Acad Dermatol. 1999;41(6):911–4.
28. Bingham JS. Carcinoma of the penis developed in lichen sclerosus et atrophicus. Br J Vener Dis. 1978;54(5):350–1.
29. Mikhail GR. Cancers, precancers and pseudocancers of the male genitalia: a review of clinical appearances, histopathology, and management. J Dermatol Surg Oncol. 1980;6:1027–35.
30. Powell J, Robson A, Cranston D, et al. High incidence of lichen sclerosus in patients with squamous cell carcinoma of the penis. Br J Dermatol. 2001;145:85–9.
31. Fergus KB, Lee AW, Baradaran N, Cohen AJ, Stohr BA, Erickson BA, Mmonu NA, Breyer BN. Pathophysiology, clinical manifestations, and treatment of lichen Sclerosus: a systematic review. Urology. 2020;135:11–9.
32. Lewis FM, Tatnall FM, Velangi SS, et al. British Association of Dermatologists guidelines for the management of lichen sclerosus, 2018. Br J Dermatol. 2018;178:839–53.
33. Depasquale I, Park AJ, Bracka A. The treatment of balanitis xerotica obliterans. BJU Int. 2000;
34. Morey AF, Lin HC, DeRosa CA, Griffith BC. Fossa navicularis reconstruction: impact of stricture length on outcomes and assessment of extended meatotomy (first stage Johanson) maneuver. J Urol. 2007;177:184–7.
35. Kim JY, Kim JY, Park M, et al. Surgical managements of pseudoepitheliomatous keratotic and micaceous balanitis: a case report. Int J Surg Case Rep. 2019;55:37–40.
36. Spencer A, Watchorn RE, Kravvas G, Ben-Salha I, Haider A, Francis N, Freeman A, Alnajjar HM, Muneer A, Bunker CB. Pseudoepitheliomatous keratotic and micaceous balanitis: a series of eight cases. J Eur Acad Dermatol Venereol. 2022;36(10):1851–6.
37. Lowe FC, McCullough AR. Cutaneous horns of the penis: an approach to management. Case report and review of the literature. J Am Acad Dermatol. 1985;13:369–73.
38. Eaglstein WH, Weinstein GD, Frost P. Fluorouracil: mechanism of action in human skin and actinic keratoses. I. Effect on DNA synthesis in vivo. Arch Dermatol. 1970;101(2):132–9.
39. Goette DK, Carson TE. Erythroplasia of Queyrat: treatment with topical 5-fluorouracil. Cancer. 1976;38(4):1498–502. https://doi.org/10.1002/1097-0142(197610)38:4<1498::aid-cncr2820380409>3.0.co;2-#.
40. Goette DK, Elgart M, DeVillez RL. Erythroplasia of Queyrat. Treatment with topically applied fluorouracil. JAMA. 1975;232(9):934–7. https://doi.org/10.1001/jama.232.9.934.
41. Alnajjar HM, Lam W, Bolgeri M, Rees RW, Perry MJ, Watkin NA. Treatment of carcinoma in situ of the glans penis with topical chemotherapy agents. Eur Urol. 2012;62(5):923–8. https://doi.org/10.1016/j.eururo.2012.02.052.
42. Issa A, Sebro K, Kwok A, et al. Treatment options and outcomes for men with penile intraepithelial neoplasia: a systematic review [published online ahead of print, 2021 may 11]. Eur Urol Focus. 2021.;S2405-4569(21)00132-2; https://doi.org/10.1016/j.euf.2021.04.026.
43. Hegarty PK, Shabbir M, Hughes B, et al. Penile preserving surgery and surgical strategies to maximize penile form and function in penile cancer: recommendations from the

United Kingdom experience. World J Urol. 2009;27(2):179–87. https://doi.org/10.1007/s00345-008-0312-x.

44. Hengge UR, Benninghoff B, Ruzicka T, Goos M. Topical immunomodulators--progress towards treating inflammation, infection, and cancer [published correction appears in Lancet Infect Dis 2002 Apr;2(4):259]. Lancet Infect Dis. 2001;1(3):189–98. https://doi.org/10.1016/s1473-3099(01)00095-0.
45. Deen K, Burdon-Jones D. Imiquimod in the treatment of penile intraepithelial neoplasia: an update. Australas J Dermatol. 2017;58(2):86–92. https://doi.org/10.1111/ajd.12466.
46. Baust JG, Gage AA. The molecular basis of cryosurgery. BJU Int. 2005;95(9):1187–91. https://doi.org/10.1111/j.1464-410X.2005.05502.x.
47. Hansen JP, Drake AL, Walling HW. Bowen's disease: a four-year retrospective review of epidemiology and treatment at a university center. Dermatol Surg. 2008;34(7):878–83. https://doi.org/10.1111/j.1524-4725.2008.34172.x.
48. Shaw KS, Nguyen GH, Lacouture M, Deng L. Combination of imiquimod with cryotherapy in the treatment of penile intraepithelial neoplasia. JAAD Case Rep. 2017;3(6):546–9. Published 2017 Nov 6. https://doi.org/10.1016/j.jdcr.2017.07.018.
49. Bandieramonte G, Colecchia M, Mariani L, et al. Peniscopically controlled CO2 laser excision for conservative treatment of in situ and T1 penile carcinoma: report on 224 patients. Eur Urol. 2008;54(4):875–82. https://doi.org/10.1016/j.eururo.2008.01.019.
50. Chipollini J, Yan S, Ottenhof SR, et al. Surgical management of penile carcinoma in situ: results from an international collaborative study and review of the literature. BJU Int. 2018;121(3):393–8. https://doi.org/10.1111/bju.14037.
51. Meijer RP, Boon TA, van Venrooij GE, Wijburg CJ. Long-term follow-up after laser therapy for penile carcinoma. Urology. 2007;69(4):759–62. https://doi.org/10.1016/j.urology.2007.01.023.
52. Schlenker B, Tilki D, Seitz M, et al. Organ-preserving neodymium-yttrium-aluminium-garnet laser therapy for penile carcinoma: a long-term follow-up. BJU Int. 2010;106(6):786–90. https://doi.org/10.1111/j.1464-410X.2009.09188.x.
53. Frimberger D, Hungerhuber E, Zaak D, Waidelich R, Hofstetter A, Schneede P. Penile carcinoma. Is Nd:YAG laser therapy radical enough? J Urol. 2002;168(6):2418–21. https://doi.org/10.1097/01.ju.0000036629.28231.85.
54. Maranda EL, Nguyen AH, Lim VM, Shah VV, Jimenez JJ. Erythroplasia of Queyrat treated by laser and light modalities: a systematic review. Lasers Med Sci. 2016;31(9):1971–6. https://doi.org/10.1007/s10103-016-2005-9. Epub 2016 Jun 21
55. Mohs F, Snow S, Larson P. Mohs micrographic surgery for penile tumours. Urol Clin North Am. 1992;19:291–304.
56. Shindel A, Mann M, Lev R, et al. Mohs micrographic surgery for penile cancer: management and long-term follow-up. J Urol. 2007;178:1980–5.
57. Depasquale I, Park A, Brack A. The treatment of balanitis xerotica obliterans. BJU Int. 2000;86:459–65.
58. Hadway P, Corbishley C, Watkin N. Total glans resurfacing for premalignant lesions of the penis: initial outcome data. BJU Int. 2006;98:532–6.
59. Shabbir M, Muneer A, Kalsi J, et al. Glans resurfacing for the treatment of carcinoma in situ of the penis: surgical technique and outcomes. Eur Urol. 2011;59:142–7.
60. O'Kelly F, Lonergan P, Lundon D, et al. A prospective study of total glans resurfacing for localised penile cancer to maximize oncological and functional ouctomes in a tertiary referral network. J Urol. 2017;197:1258–63.
61. Ayres B, Al-Najjar H, Corbishley C, Perry M, Watkin N. Oncological outcomes of glans resurfacing in the treatment of selected superficially invasive penile cancers. J Urol. 2012;187(Suppl 4):e306.
62. Malone PR, Thomas JS, Blick C. A tie-over dressing for graft application in distal penectomy and glans resurfacing: the TODGA technique. BJU Int. 2011;107(5):836–40.
63. Cakir OO, Schifano N, Venturino L, Pozzi E, Castiglione F, Alnajjar HM, Muneer A. Surgical technique and outcomes following coronal-sparing glans resurfacing for benign and malignant penile lesions. Int J Impot Res. 2022;34(5):495–500.

6 Penile-Sparing Surgical Options for Patients Diagnosed with Penile Cancer

James A. Churchill and Vijay K. Sangar

Learning Objectives
After reading this chapter you will be able to:

- Describe the relevant anatomy for the surgical management of penile cancer
- Discuss penile-sparing surgical options for local control of penile cancer depending on the location and stage of disease
- Summarise important considerations for pre-operative patient preparation and counselling
- Understand the techniques and post-operative care for penile-sparing surgical management options, including circumcision, glansectomy (total and partial) and wide local excision.

Introduction

The principles of surgical management of penile cancer are [1] oncologic control, by safe excision of the primary tumour with an adequate margin, and [2] preservation of sexual function, urinary function, and quality of life (QOL) using reconstructive techniques. The surgical procedures and techniques required for comprehensive cancer care are heavily influenced by the location of the tumour and the extent to which the tumour has invaded adjacent tissues. This chapter describes penile sparing surgical treatments available for penile cancer localised to the prepuce (foreskin), glans and penile shaft.

J. A. Churchill · V. K. Sangar (✉)
The Christie NHS Foundation Trust, Manchester, UK
e-mail: vijay.sangar@nhs.net

O. Brunckhorst et al. (eds.), *Penile Cancer – A Practical Guide*, Management of Urology, https://doi.org/10.1007/978-3-031-32681-3_6

Anatomy

The basic but important anatomical features relevant to localised penile cancer surgery include the relationship of the prepuce, Buck's fascia, neurovascular bundle, glans, corpus spongiosum and corpora cavernosa. Figure 3.1 shows a cross-section of the penis to demonstrate the proximity of these structures.

The AJCC TNM staging system [2] is described in detail in Chap. 4, but briefly, defines T1 tumours as those invading subepithelial connective tissue with subclassification into T1a and T1b depending on lymphovascular invasion and differentiation status, T2 tumours as those invading corpus spongiosum and T3 tumours as those invading corpora cavernosa. Notably, the TNM staging system is periodically updated [3]. Relevant to this chapter, stage specifications were revised in 2010 such that urethral involvement was replaced with corpora cavernosa involvement as the differentiating factor between T2 and T3. Caution should therefore be used when reviewing histopathology reports or the literature prior to 2010, as the staging system referenced may not be current.

In addition to staging considerations, Buck's fascia is an important anatomical structure to recognise for its use in supporting grafted tissue during reconstruction. Intraoperatively, a dissection 'over' Buck's fascia is notable for the presence of vessels on its overlying surface, whereas a dissection 'under' Buck's fascia leaves a relatively avascular tunica albuginea.

Imaging for primary tumours may be performed where findings will change management, as may be the case for glans tumours with suspected corpora cavernosa involvement but where maximum preservation of penile length is desired, and in cases of suspected skip lesions or recurrence. Options for imaging are covered extensively in Chap. 3 but include penile MRI, with artificial erection by intracavernosal injection or doppler US to evaluate corpora cavernosa involvement [4, 5].

Choice of Procedure

The surgical procedure indicated for treatment of the primary tumour depends on the location and T-stage, as described in Fig. 6.1.

Procedures may be grouped into penile-sparing surgery (circumcision, wide local excision and partial/total glansectomy) and non-penile sparing surgery (partial/total penectomy). Other penile-sparing techniques, such as laser ablation, glans resurfacing and Mohs micrographic surgery, are well described for penile intraepithelial neoplasia (and may be appropriate for low-risk T1 tumours) but are covered in further detail in Chap. 5. This chapter will be focussing on the penile-sparing surgical options described above.

One challenge of penile cancer management is that initial diagnosis is often by clinical examination and with limited histological confirmation. Shave, punch or incisional biopsies, whereby larger lesions are sampled, can confirm a diagnosis, and may demonstrate the grade accurately, but do not adequately define the T-stage which is often under-staged. Final T-stage is often not confirmed until after a

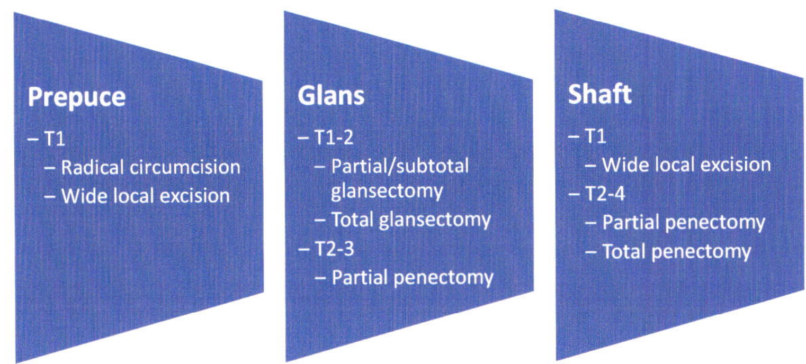

Fig. 6.1 Surgical procedure options by tumour location and T-stage

definitive penile cancer procedure, underlining the importance of a detailed clinical examination to determine the extent of local invasion.

Prepuce

Tumours on the prepuce can be treated by performing a radical circumcision, where a negative margin is achievable with minimal morbidity.

Glans

Tumours on the glans clinically staged as T1 or T2 generally require glansectomy, whether partial or total. Glans resurfacing, which is indicated for PeIN and covered in Chap. 10 of this book, may be performed for selected patients with low volume and low-risk T1(a) tumours. Where a tumour is small (<1–2 cm depending on the exact location), a negative margin is achievable and where the remaining glans will not present significant deformity or deviation of the urethra, a partial/subtotal glansectomy is suitable and may allow the patient to retain function in the remaining glans. Lesions which are located on the glans corona can be excised with the foreskin and an advancement flap of shaft skin can cover the partial glans defect. Total glansectomy is indicated where a tumour occupies a sufficient area of the glans such that a negative margin is not achievable, where partial glansectomy will lead to glans deformity and/or urethral deviation and generally where a tumour involves the distal urethra (within the glans).

Shaft

Tumours on the shaft that are mobile (clinical T1) may be managed with wide local excision, with or without scrotal advancement flaps to ensure tension-free closure to accommodate future erections. The guidance on the tumour-free distance required for an adequate surgical margin has evolved, with current guidelines recommending a risk-adapted strategy of 3–8 mm based on the tumour grade [6].

Skin flap and split thickness skin graft (STSG) techniques are often used in combination with many of these procedures to reconstruct a neoglans and improve the cosmetic outcome. Urethral reconstruction is required for procedures that excise the urethra, including glansectomy, partial and total penectomy. This may be performed by simple spatulation and formation of a neo-meatus when penile-sparing surgery is performed, but both subtotal and total penectomy require urinary diversion in the form of a perineal urethrostomy.

Counselling and Consent

The selection of surgical treatment for penile cancer should be undertaken through assessment and shared decision-making between clinician and patient, acknowledging the oncologic benefits, procedural risks, and functional outcomes of available treatments.

As with any medical consent process, informed consent requires a competent patient who is able to understand, retain and make an informed choice based on presentation of risks, benefits, and alternatives for the proposed course of treatment, including the implications of no treatment at all. Material risks will differ for each patient, but generally include the peri-procedure, early and late complications. The patient should understand the expected oncologic and functional outcomes, including the indications for further investigations and treatment.

Disease-specific patient information sheets and adjunct consultations with specialist nursing staff recommended during the assessment and consent phases. The British Association of Urological Surgeons (BAUS) produces excellent national-standard information sheets on penile cancer procedures for those based in the United Kingdom [7], which may either be provided directly or adapted to the local context.

Thorough pre-operative assessment is important for penile cancer patients, who tend to be older with multiple medical co-morbidities. Careful elucidation of capacity and performance status is recommended, and anaesthetic risks may be reduced by pre-operative optimisation and education. Anticoagulants should generally be withheld in the pre-operative period, except aspirin in those at highest cardiac thrombotic risk, as the glans and corpora cavernosa are highly vascular structures. Notably, all the penile procedures described in this chapter (except split-thickness skin grafts (STSG)) are suitable to perform under spinal anaesthetic and a surprising number under local anaesthetic (LA), with an appropriately consented patient and an effective local anaesthetic penile block.

Preparation

All procedures below assume an appropriately consented and informed patient with completion of WHO surgical timeout processes, IV antibiotic prophylaxis (as per local guidance) and VTE prophylaxis, in the supine position with all pressure areas attended.

Most of procedures require a number 11 or 15 scalpel, bipolar diathermy, 4-0 and 5/0 absorbable sutures and a general or plastics instrument set. Though the number 15 scalpel is an accepted standard for dermato-surgical skin incisions, an 11-blade is also well suited to fine incisions, as may be required for partial glansectomy or wide local excisions. A penile tourniquet is required for glansectomy and partial penectomy, which is readily available as an elastic Penrose drain or vessel loop with small forceps used for application.

A penile block provides excellent analgesia for any operation of the penis and should routinely be performed at the start of the procedure, even if the patient is under general anaesthesia. Plain anaesthetic agent (without adrenaline) with a 22G (blue) needle should be injected at the base of the penis under the pubic arch, the depth of which varies greatly on body habitus. As the dorsal nerves branch extensively in this location, inject in an area 1–2 cm either side of the midline.

Circumcision

Technique

A circumcision is the starting point for many penile cancer procedures. Mark all planned incisions and the midline on the ventral shaft skin, with sufficient skin remaining to accommodate a fully erect penis (measured on stretch).

There are several techniques described for circumcision with the following recommended for adult 'radical' circumcision for penile cancer treatment. The first step is often to perform a dorsal slit to permit retraction if required by a tight phimosis, though preferably do not incise through tumour and (as always with a dorsal slit) take care to avoid the urethral meatus. Division of any glans adhesions can be performed with tenotomy scissors.

Place a mosquito clip on the penile shaft skin parallel to the corona at 12 o'clock, a mosquito clip at 6 o'clock and a further 2 mosquito clips at the 3 and 9 o'clock positions on the prepuce to allow effective tension. Incise the outer prepuce and dartos in an oblique line between the 6 and 12 o'clock clips. Retract the prepuce and incise the frenulum with a circumcoronal inner prepuce incision about 5 mm from the coronal border (or closer if required by tumour), controlling vessels and to a depth that allows visualisation of Buck's fascia. Complete the dorsal slit through the inner and outer prepuce to the level of circumcoronal incision. The prepuce can be dissected together with the tumour and the specimen should be orientated and marked for pathological review. Closure with 4/0 and 5/0 absorbable sutures can be performed followed by application of a dry dressing.

Post-Operative Care

Discharge patients on the day of surgery when voiding (nurse-led) with instructions to remove the dressing on day 1. Cases should be referred to a specialist multidisciplinary meeting. It is worthwhile advising patients that cosmetic appearances of a newly circumcised penis improve over the first 6 weeks after operation.

Glansectomy

Technique

A total glansectomy starts with a circumferential outer skin incision as for a circumcision. If previously circumcised, complete this at the site of the previous circumcision scar. Deepen this circumferentially until a well-vascularised layer of Dartos fascia is seen to cover Buck's fascia. Consider a penile tourniquet if a partial penectomy is required.

Perform a dissection 'over' Buck's fascia to preserve the vascular supply to the graft. Develop a plane between Buck's fascia and the glans and dissect distally using tenotomy scissors, using both sharp and blunt dissection. Continue until the urethra is the only remaining attachment, maintaining 1 cm length beyond the corpora cavernosa if possible.

In cases where a STSG is not required, and particularly with tumours that are adherent to the Bucks' fascia a dissection 'under' Buck's fascia is preferred. This begins with a clear definition of the urethra; consider temporary placement of a 14Fr catheter to aid this. Make two parallel 3–4 mm longitudinal incisions either side of urethra through Buck's fascia and deepen with the blade until the tunica albuginea is visualised. Take care not to incise through the tunica albuginea and into the corpora cavernosa. The dorsal neurovascular bundle can be identified and ligated and dissection continues under the Bucks' fascia and glans leaving the tunica albuginea intact.

Transect the urethra with a clean scalpel at a slightly oblique angle, longer at the dorsal aspect. If any doubt regarding surgical margin exists, take shave biopsies from each corpora cavernosa tip to send for histopathology. Spatulate the ventral aspect of the urethra for 1–1.5 cm and splay this over the corpora cavernosa heads at 2–4 points with 4-0 absorbable sutures. Bring the skin to the urethra with a 4-0 absorbable suture, with attention to the (proximal) apex of the spatulated urethra. Place a 14Fr 2-way indwelling catheter (IDC) and dress with paraffin lattice, light gauze and crepe/elastic bandage.

Partial/Subtotal Variations

A partial or subtotal glansectomy technique is dependent on tumour location, size, depth and proximity to the urethra and corpora cavernosa. The principles are of complete tumour removal with preservation of part of the glans, while achieving adequate surgical margins (3–8 mm). The tissues of most interest in preservation are the peri-urethral tissues and the corona. Therefore, the most amenable lesions are those at the glans periphery where a section of glans tissue may be excised whilst preserving the urethra, peri-urethral glans, and remaining corona. Consideration should be given to how the asymmetrically resected glans will affect urinary and sexual function, and whether oncological and functional goals may be better served by performing a total glansectomy.

As the glans is highly vascular structure, a penile tourniquet is recommended for all but the smallest of partial glansectomies, to allow for maximum visualisation of the tissue being excised. A positive margin at partial glansectomy usually necessitates a completion glansectomy at a later date.

In an uncircumcised patient, a circumcision will be required, and outer preputial skin or shaft skin can be marked as a template to cover the glans defect created by excising the tumour. In a previously circumcised patient, skin reconstruction after a partial glansectomy is usually facilitated by an advancement flap of shaft skin (see section below). In both cases, vertical mattress sutures are recommended when bringing skin to a cut glans surface, with deep suture passes serving dual roles to reinforce a tissue closure of edges at uneven levels and to ensure glans haemostasis.

The patient should be counselled that an advancement flap may become asymmetrically 'tight' with erections and, particularly in cases where the initial circumcision has left insufficient skin.

A specific variant on this technique is a coronal-sparing glansectomy, whereby a central tumour is excised (with urethral meatus) preserving the entire of the corona. A skin graft may be required to cover any glans skin defect not filled by the reconstructed urethral meatus.

Post-op Care

Patients can be discharged on the day of or day after surgery, when well and catheter-educated, with instructions to remove the penile dressing on day 1 and return for a TWOC on day 5–7. Patients after larger partial glansectomy procedures may warrant observation overnight, for confirmation of tissue viability in the remaining glans on day 1.

Wide Local Excision (WLE)

Technique

The technique for this procedure is reliant on the location and size of tumour. Deep tumours involving the corpora spongiosum (cT2) or cavernosa (cT3) are unsuitable for a WLE, and occasionally a clinically under-staged tumour planned for WLE requires intraoperative conversion to a glansectomy or partial penectomy.

Start with either a penile block or, if the lesion is close to the base of the penis where innervation may extend from the pre-pubic skin, consider direct LA infiltration but keep in mind that tissue planes are often distorted by the injected fluid volume. Excise the lesion sharply with usual guidance on margins (3–8 mm) and with consideration of closure of the incision parallel to skin tension lines (i.e. Langer's lines). In general, a transverse incision is preferred to a longitudinal one due to a lower risk of skin cicatrisation (narrowing). Achieve haemostasis with bipolar diathermy and close with 3-0 or 4-0 absorbable sutures depending on the location and required tensile strength. If wide local excision will result in a primary skin closure under tension in the fully erect penis, a local skin flap or skin graft will be required (see below).

Skin Flaps/Grafts

Indications

A skin flap or graft is indicated where a skin defect resulting from any of the above procedures cannot be primarily closed without tension in the fully erect penis, particularly where a previous procedure has created a pre-existing shortage of available skin. Where a foreskin is available, it can often be used creatively to minimise the need for flap/graft reconstruction.

The functional consequences of penile skin tension can be significant, with bothersome pain and tethering/curvature on erection—only in cases of severe erectile dysfunction can this risk be discounted.

Skin flaps are preferred where available skin can be mobilised to cover a defect with minimal additional intervention. An advancement flap is generally the simplest means of gaining additional skin for lesions of the distal penile shaft and glans, whereby shaft skin is undermined over Buck's fascia for 1–4 cm proximally and brought up to cover the defect. Keep in mind that the width of the flap may need to be substantially wider than the width of the defect, to allow for adequate mobility and cosmesis.

A STSG is a versatile technique for covering defects of the glans and shaft but is associated with morbidity – donor sites tend to be much more painful than recipient sites—and the risk of complications include graft loss [8]. As the split skin takes the blood supply of the tissue over which it is grafted, caution should be exercised with current smokers (or those who have quit less than 6 weeks ago) and those with diabetes. Success or failure of a penile skin graft is a powerful motivation to quit smoking.

Technique

Complete the required excision, place a urethral catheter, ensuring that the donor and recipient site are free from contamination. Use a dermatome to harvest a STSG from the thigh, with a suggested thickness of 0.0016 inches and dimensions suitable to cover the area of the defect. We use an air-driven Zimmer dermatome, but other models produce similar results. The side that the graft is taken may be chosen either by the handedness of the patient or of the surgeon. Place the graft flat on the back of a plastic kidney dish, with skin surface facing up and dermal (shiny) surface facing down. Infiltrate the donor site with 10mls of lignocaine 1% with adrenaline and dress with alginate-based dressing under a large plastic film dressing.

Our preference is not to perforate the graft, but we recognise that this is a common practice and may provide an opportunity for entrapped blood to escape in the immediate post-operative period. Before placing the graft, re-examine the recipient site for haemostasis, balancing the need for healthy vascular supply for the graft with the avoidance of haematoma formation and separation of graft from underlying tissues. In practice, a light venous ooze is tolerated, but arterial bleeding must be controlled.

Tailor the graft to the required area and fix to the recipient site using 5-0 absorbable suture, always placing sutures first through the delicate graft. The technique of placing multiple sutures and then 'parachuting' the graft down is particularly graceful. We have recently commenced using Artiss Sealant skin glue [9] injected under the graft to aid adherence between the graft and underlying tissue, with excellent early graft function and short length of stay (data pending publication). Apply gentle pressure to the graft using a wet swab while a tie-over 'TODGA' dressing is prepared and applied [10]. We use a paraffin lattice folded 10-times over, trimmed in a horse-shoe shape to permit the passage of the urethral catheter if needed and secured with 3-0 non-absorbable suture through skin (adjacent to graft) and multiple layers of dressing in a tie-over pattern that allows for atraumatic removal.

Post-op Care

Post-op plans are as per the primary operation, plus re-dressing of donor site on day 1 and broad-spectrum antibiotic for 5 days. The patient should not remove dressings, shower or bath until the tie-over dressing and catheter are removed on day 7, at which point re-application of a non-adherent dressing may be needed if areas of the graft are slow to take.

Complications and Side Effects

When discussing risks of penile operations, the framework of general and specific, early, and late complications is valid. General complications of anaesthesia including cardiorespiratory compromise, venous thromboembolism and anaesthetic reaction should be discussed, alongside early specific complications of bleeding, infection, and discomfort. Below, we discuss the oncologic and functional late complications of surgery for localised penile cancer.

Oncologic Outcomes

The primary oncologic risk/outcome measure of surgery for primary penile tumours is the recurrence rate. In penile sparing surgery (defined as circumcision, partial/total glansectomy, WLE, laser ablation and glans resurfacing) is associated with a 20–27% risk of recurrence, with a positive margin associated with an increased risk of local recurrence [11, 12].

Despite the increased risk of local recurrence with penile sparing surgery, five-year cancer-specific survival is similar in patients treated with partial penectomy and penile-sparing surgery [11, 13, 14], supporting the use of penile-sparing surgery. However, more recent data indicate that pathological T3 stage and higher-grade disease are associated with increased risk of local recurrence after glansectomy and that such recurrence has a worse overall and cancer-specific survival, indicating aggressive disease and challenging the role of penile sparing surgery [15]. It is critical that the patient is educated and motivated to self-examine during follow-up, to support early detection of recurrence [6].

Functional and QOL Outcomes

Literature on the sexual function, urinary function, and quality of life (QOL) outcomes after penile cancer surgery is sparse but is covered in more detail in Chap. 11 of this book. Broadly, penile cancer treatment may have an impact on sexual function, quality of life (QOL), social interactions, self-image, and self-esteem, with up to 40% reporting negative wellbeing effects [16]. Men tend to report greater impact on sexual function with partial penectomy than penile-sparing surgery [17] and with glansectomy than WLE [18], validating a penile-sparing approach from the perspective of sexual function outcomes. Urinary function is not well studied, but risks of any operation that involves resection of the urethra include stenosis and spraying. Loss of length may result in the patient requiring the use of a funnel and/or sitting to pass urine, particularly with partial penectomy in which 83% report leakage, compared with 43% after penile-sparing surgery [17].

Key Points

- The relationship of a tumour to penile anatomical structures (corpus spongiosum, corpora cavernosa) defines the clinical T-stage and must be carefully considered for effective operative planning and patient counselling
- Penile-sparing surgical options for excision of clinical T1-2 penile tumours include circumcision, wide local excision and partial/total glansectomy.
- Choice of operation depends on the location and depth of tissue invasion.
- Patient counselling and shared decision-making is important given the oncologic, functional and QOL outcomes of surgery for penile tumours

Revision Questions

Multiple Choice Questions

1. When assessing local stage in penile cancer, which of the following is not routinely used?
   A. Ultrasound of the penis and inguinal regions
   B. Clinical examination

   C. Incision or punch biopsy of lesion
   D. MRI
2. In assessing a patient for treatment of a T1-2 penile cancer, which of these would likely be a suitable operation:
   A. Glansectomy and split thickness graft reconstruction
   B. Partial penectomy
   C. Circumcision
   D. CO2 laser ablation
3. When performing a skin graft procedure with penile surgery, which type of skin graft is normally utilised?
   A. Hairy full thickness graft
   B. Mohs thickness graft
   C. Hairless full thickness graft
   D. Hairless split thickness graft

Viva Cases

Case 1

A 59-year-old gentleman presents with a six-month history of enlarging penile mass (Fig. 6.2).

A. How would you assess this gentleman?
B. In what scenario would you perform further local staging imaging for this patient?
C. From examination and investigations, you determine that this tumour is clinical T2 confined to the glans. Which operation would you recommend for this gentleman and justify why?

Answers

Multiple Choice Questions

1. **C.** Biopsy of a lesion will usually only provide a diagnosis and grade of malignancy (if present). It will not provide local stage, as it only samples part of the lesion.
2. **A.** A patient with a T1-2 tumour confined to the glans should undergo glansectomy and would likely result in a negative margin, as the tumour would not breach the plane beneath the glans penis. Circumcision would be undertaken as part of the procedure but would not remove the tumour itself. Laser ablation is not suitable for invasive tumours. Partial penectomy would allow excision of the glans and a section of corpora cavernosa with a negative margin, however, will lead to an unnecessarily shorter penis and inferior cosmetic and functional outcomes.

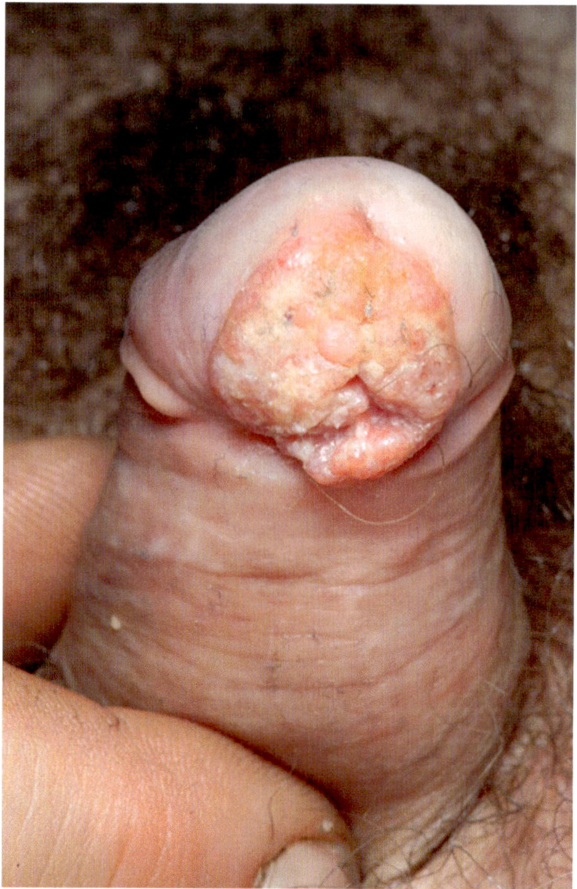

Fig. 6.2 Penile squamous cell carcinoma. Image courtesy of Mr. Arie Parnham

3. **D**. Hairless skin is always used, for better cosmesis and function. Split-thickness skin grafts are best as they allow better uptake of blood supply from the penile bed and/or Bucks fascia than full-thickness skin grafts.

Viva Cases

Case 1

A. Take a focussed urological history including:
   - Symptoms and chronology
   - Effect on sexual and urinary function
   - Systemic features of malignancy (lymphadenopathy, weight loss etc)
   - Penile cancer risk factors
   - Co-morbidities
   - Medications

- Social history
- Perform an examination (chaperoned) including:
- Body habitus including abdominal/pre-pubic fat depth
- Key penile anatomical structures involved by the tumour to assess extent of invasion, specifically noting urethral and corpora cavernosa involvement
- Length of normal external penile shaft remaining below palpable extent of lesion
- Bilateral inguinal examination noting number, site, size and character (fixation) of any palpable lymph nodes
- Perineum and proximal corpora cavernosa to ensure that no evidence of scrotal or bone extension or skip lesions

B. Perform local staging imaging where findings will change management. In this case, an MRI would only be reasonable if corpora cavernosa invasion is suspected, however clinical examination may be able to exclude this here.

C. This gentleman would be able to undergo a partial glansectomy with a split-thickness skin graft as a suitable penile-sparing option. The aim is to be able to achieve excision of the tumour while achieving adequate surgical margins (3–8 mm) while trying to preserve functional and quality of life outcomes. However, if this margin is not believed to be achieved, if resection would leave a largely asymmetrical glans (which will affect urinary/sexual function), or if a positive margin occurs a total glansectomy would be required.

Acknowledgements The authors of the chapter would like to thank Mr. Arie Parnham for his help with the figures for this chapter.

Test your learning and check your understanding of this book's contents: use the "Springer Nature Flashcards" app to access questions using ▶ https://sn.pub/1r7Om8. To use the app, please follow the instructions in chapter 1.

References

1. MacLennan G. Penis and male urethra. In: Hinman's Atlas of UroSurgical Anatomy. 2nd Edition. Elsevier; 2012. p. 305–34.
2. Amin MB, Edge SB, Greene FL, Byrd DR, Brookland RK, Washington MK, et al., editors. AJCC cancer staging manual. 8th ed. Springer Cham; 2017. 1032 p.
3. Paner GP, Stadler WM, Hansel DE, Montironi R, Lin DW, Amin MB. Updates in the eighth edition of the tumor-node-metastasis staging classification for urologic cancers. Eur Urol. 2018;73(4):560–9.
4. Hanchanale V, Yeo L, Subedi N, Smith J, Wah T, Harnden P, et al. The accuracy of magnetic resonance imaging (MRI) in predicting the invasion of the tunica albuginea and the urethra during the primary staging of penile cancer. BJU Int. 2016;117(3):439–43.
5. Bozzini G, Provenzano M, Otero JR, Margreiter M, Cruz EG, Osmolorskij B, et al. Role of penile doppler US in the preoperative assessment of penile squamous cell carcinoma patients: results from a large prospective Multicenter European Study. Urology. 2016;90:131–5.

6. Hakenberg OW, Comperat E, Minhas S, Necchi A, Protzel C, Watkin N. EAU Guidelines on Penile Cancer. 2018 Mar p. 1 37. (EAU Guidelines).
7. British Association of Urological Surgeons. Penis procedures [Internet]. [cited 2022 Apr 10]. Available from: https://www.baus.org.uk/patients/information_leaflets/category/7/penis_procedures
8. Parnham AS, Albersen M, Sahdev V, Christodoulidou M, Nigam R, Malone P, et al. Glansectomy and split-thickness skin graft for penile cancer. Eur Urol. 2018;73(2):284–9.
9. Boccara D, Runz AD, Bekara F, Chaouat M, Mimoun M. Artiss Sealant®. J Burn Care Res. 2017;38(5):283–9.
10. Malone PR, Thomas JS, Blick C. A tie-over dressing for graft application in distal penectomy and glans resurfacing: the TODGA technique. BJU Int. 2010;107(5):836–40.
11. Djajadiningrat RS, Werkhoven E van, Meinhardt W, van Rhijn BWG, Bex A, van der Poel HG, et al. Penile sparing surgery for penile cancer—does it affect survival? J Urol 2014;192(1):120–126.
12. Baumgarten A, Chipollini J, Yan S, Ottenhof SR, Tang DH, Draeger D, et al. Penile sparing surgery for penile cancer: a multicenter international retrospective cohort. J Urol. 2018;199(5):1233–7.
13. Leijte JAP, Kirrander P, Antonini N, Windahl T, Horenblas S. Recurrence patterns of squamous cell carcinoma of the penis: recommendations for follow-up based on a two-centre analysis of 700 patients. Eur Urol. 2008;54(1):161–9.
14. Kamel MH, Bissada N, Warford R, Farias J, Davis R. Organ sparing surgery for penile cancer: a systematic review. J Urol. 2017;198(4):770–9.
15. Roussel E, Peeters E, Vanthoor J, Bozzini G, Muneer A, Ayres B, et al. Predictors of local recurrence and its impact on survival after glansectomy for penile cancer: time to challenge the dogma? BJU Int. 2021;127(5):606–13.
16. Maddineni SB, Lau MM, Sangar VK. Identifying the needs of penile cancer sufferers: a systematic review of the quality of life, psychosexual and psychosocial literature in penile cancer. BMC Urol. 2009;9(1):8–8.
17. Kieffer JM, Djajadiningrat RS, van Muilekom EAM, Graafland NM, Horenblas S, Aaronson NK. Quality of life for patients treated for penile cancer. J Urol. 2014;192(4):1105–10.
18. Sedigh O, Falcone M, Ceruti C, Timpano M, Preto M, Oderda M, et al. Sexual function after surgical treatment for penile cancer: which organ-sparing approach gives the best results? Can Urol Assoc J. 2015;9(7–8):423–7.

Surgical Management of Advanced Penile Cancer

7

Yao Zhu, Dingwei Ye, and Weijie Gu

Learning Objectives
After reading this chapter you will be able to:

- Describe the surgical management options for advanced penile cancer, including partial and total penectomy
- Summarise the operative management of patients with pelvic lymph node metastasis
- Review common complications arising from the surgical management of advanced penile cancer

The Definition, Prognosis, and Treatment Paradigm of Locally Advanced Penile Cancer

Definition of Locally Advanced Penile Cancer

About 10–14% of patients with penile cancer are diagnosed with locally advanced primary disease in association with extensive inguinal metastases due to an aggressive histological subtype or a delayed presentation (Table 7.1). Locally advanced penile cancer can present with extension of the tumour into adjacent organs such as the prostate, rectum, and bladder as well as nearby osseous structures.

Penile squamous cell carcinoma has a predictable pattern of local and regional metastasis, and lymph node staging remains the strongest predictor of cancer specific survival. The 5-year disease-specific survival rates for patients with stage pN0,

Y. Zhu (✉) · D. Ye · W. Gu
Department of Urology, Fudan University Shanghai Cancer Center, Shanghai, China
e-mail: yaozhu09@fudan.edu.cn

O. Brunckhorst et al. (eds.), *Penile Cancer – A Practical Guide*, Management of Urology, https://doi.org/10.1007/978-3-031-32681-3_7

Table 7.1 The presentation of advanced penile cancer

	Symptoms
Bulky ulcerating tumours with intermittent bleeding	Cachexia
	Anaemia
	Fatigue
Osseous metastases	Bone Pain
	Hypercalcemia
Infection	Fever
	Fatigue

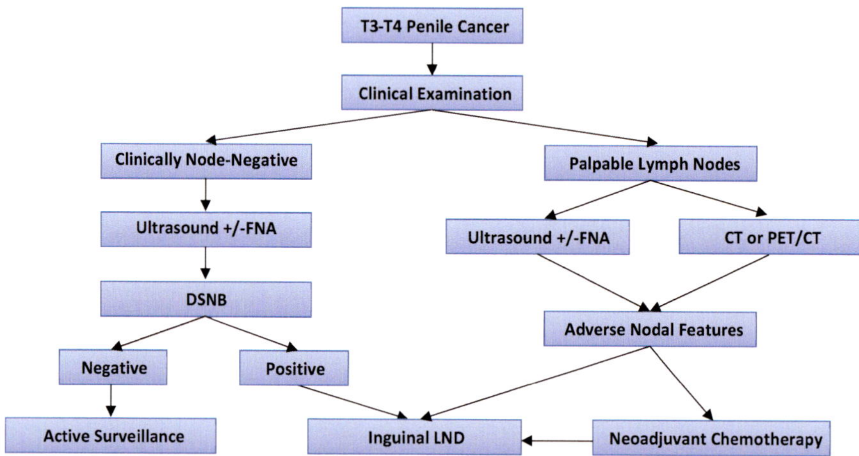

Fig. 7.1 Flow chart for management of advanced penile cancer. *FNA* fine-needle aspiration, *DSNB* dynamic sentinel node biopsy, *LND* lymph node dissection

pN1, pN2, and pN3 disease is 96%, 80%, 66%, and 37%, respectively [1]. Tumour pathologic features are also important prognostic factors, including depth of invasion, tumour grade, presence of lymphovascular invasion, and perineural invasion predicting risk of nodal spread and mortality [2–4] as previously discussed (Chap. 2).

Treatment Paradigm of Advanced Penile Cancer

Penile amputation remains the standard therapy for patients with advanced penile cancer (T3-T4). Partial or total penectomy should be considered in patients exhibiting invasive tumours which extend into the corpus cavernosum and extend proximally.

The management of regional lymph nodes is more complicated (Fig. 7.1). Resection of small volume pathologically involved regional lymph nodes can be curative, whereas patients with larger lymph node involvement typically are thought to benefit more from neoadjuvant chemotherapy followed by surgical consolidation. However, the management of inguinal lymph nodes will be covered in detail in Chap. 8.

Table 7.2 Preoperative assessment

Physical examination	Identify palpable lymph nodes
Pathology	Biopsy of suspicious lymph node
MRI	Evaluate the extension of tumour to plan the surgical management
PET-CT	Identify regional or distant metastases

Preoperative Assessment

Surgical decisions are based on the primary tumour pathological features, clinical nodal status, and imaging results (Table 7.2). More detailed information on the staging and imaging process is provided in Chaps. 3 and 4. It is important that patients with clinically palpable lymph nodes and those with high-risk primary tumours should undergo imaging to define the full extent of disease before beginning multimodal disease management.

Most patients identified to have advanced penile cancer would benefit from a multimodal treatment approach combining chemotherapy with consolidation surgical treatment as is discussed in Chap. 9.

Although no comparative studies exist on the use of pre-operative antibiotics, it seems to be rational to give prophylactic antibiotics due to coexisting infection within the lymph nodes.

Penectomy

Partial Penectomy

For patients identified to have T2 or T3 penile tumours, the aim of surgery is to ensure complete tumour resection with adequate tumour-free margins which traditionally have been defined as being 2 cm [5] but smaller margins are now acceptable. It is also important to preserve enough length of the penile shaft for optimisation of both urinary and sexual function, as well as minimise the psychological impact of surgery. Partial penectomy is considered for tumours involving the glans penis or distal penile shaft. The surgical procedure is described in detail in Chap. 6, but our approach can be summarised through the following steps:

1. Degloving with an incised corpora proximal to the tumour, to generate a "fish-mouth" appearance, which will allow horizontal closure.
2. The urethra should be left 10–15 mm longer than the corpora if the lesion is not ventral.
3. The corpora cavernosa is closed with an absorbable suture.
4. The shaft skin is subsequently used to cover the stump, leaving a 14 to 16Ch Foley catheter in situ and removed after around 1 week.
5. A split skin graft can also be used to avoid the shaft retracting.

A urethral centralisation technique has also been described which creates a neo-glans with a centralised urethra [6].

Total Penectomy

Some penile tumours extend so proximally that total penectomy combined with a perineal urethrostomy is required. This necessitates complete excision of the penis and crura. Preoperative antibiotics and thromboprophylaxis should be given, and antibiotics are usually continued for 1 week post-operatively.

Surgical procedure

1. An elliptical incision is performed around the tumour, followed by dissection through the skin and superficial fascia around the tumour. Subsequent division and ligation of the deep dorsal vein and neurovascular bundle is conducted along with the suspensory ligament.
2. A separate inverted U-shaped incision is made in the perineum for the perineal urethrostomy. This then requires the division of the superficial fascial layers and splitting of the bulbospongiosus muscles.
3. Identification of the urethra and ensuring the urethra has adequate length. The urethra is then transected and spatulated ventrally.
4. The crura are isolated with complete division of them near or onto the pubic bone. The crura are then oversewn using a 2/0 suture.
5. The skin is then sutured to the urethra using 4/0 and 5/0 sutures.
6. A 14 to 16 Ch Foley catheter is then left in situ and removed after around 1 week post-operatively. A drain is left in the perineum and in the pubic area, with a pressure dressing applied to reduce hematoma formation.

Complications

The main complication of partial penectomy is meatal stenosis. The risk can be minimised by ensuring that the urethral spatulation conducted is of an adequate length. If stenosis does occur, then revision surgery rather than repeated dilatations is preferred. Post total penectomy, wound infections are the most common complication. Urethral stenosis mainly occurs within the first 2 years following surgery [7].

The Role of Preoperative Chemotherapy in Advanced Disease

Patients with locally advanced penile cancer are at an increased risk of disease-related mortality with surgical treatment alone and are best treated using multimodal approaches as covered extensively in Chap. 9. Neoadjuvant systemic therapy for these patients is currently recommended as the preferred strategy by the NCCN and the EAU guidelines [8, 9]. Similarly, a previous phase 2 trial evaluating a

Paclitaxel + Ifosfamide + Cisplatin (TIP) regimen for patients with advanced penile carcinoma, had established neoadjuvant chemotherapy followed by consolidation surgical treatment as a good treatment option for patients with bulky lymphadenopathy in terms of time to progression and overall survival [10].

Managing Large Groin Defects

Large metastatic inguinal lymph nodes are associated with extracapsular extension (Fig. 7.2). To gain local control, the overlying skin and subcutaneous tissue must be removed simultaneously. Ideally, primary closure of the defect is performed at the same time, aided by mobilization of surrounding skin flaps. In patients with a good

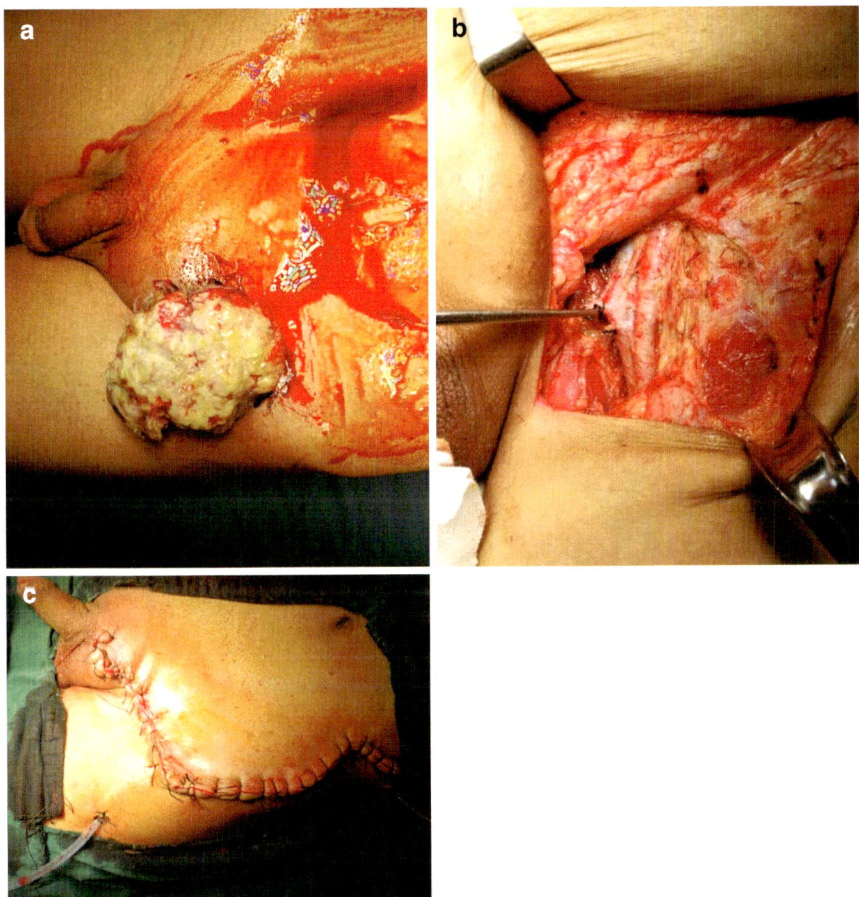

Fig. 7.2 Case 1 (**a**) Fixed and ulcerated metastatic lymph node (**b**) Complete incision of tumour and overlying skin and subcutaneous tissue (**c**) Mobilization of surrounding abdominal flap to cover the skin defect

performance status who have advanced disease, this palliative surgery provides a means to relieve pain, remove an unsightly fungating mass, and allows a better quality of life [11].

It is however worth noting that surgery alone for advanced regional penile cancer is unlikely to promote long-term survival, with a cure rate of only 27%. Moreover, it is related to a high incidence of complications. Surgical treatment with adjuvant chemotherapy is however associated with improved overall survival [12, 13].

Larger defects following resection of bulky inguinal metastatic disease are associated with skin ulceration. Therefore, these often require the use of pedicled skin flaps to cover the skin defect (Fig. 7.3). The removal of the bulky mass may again

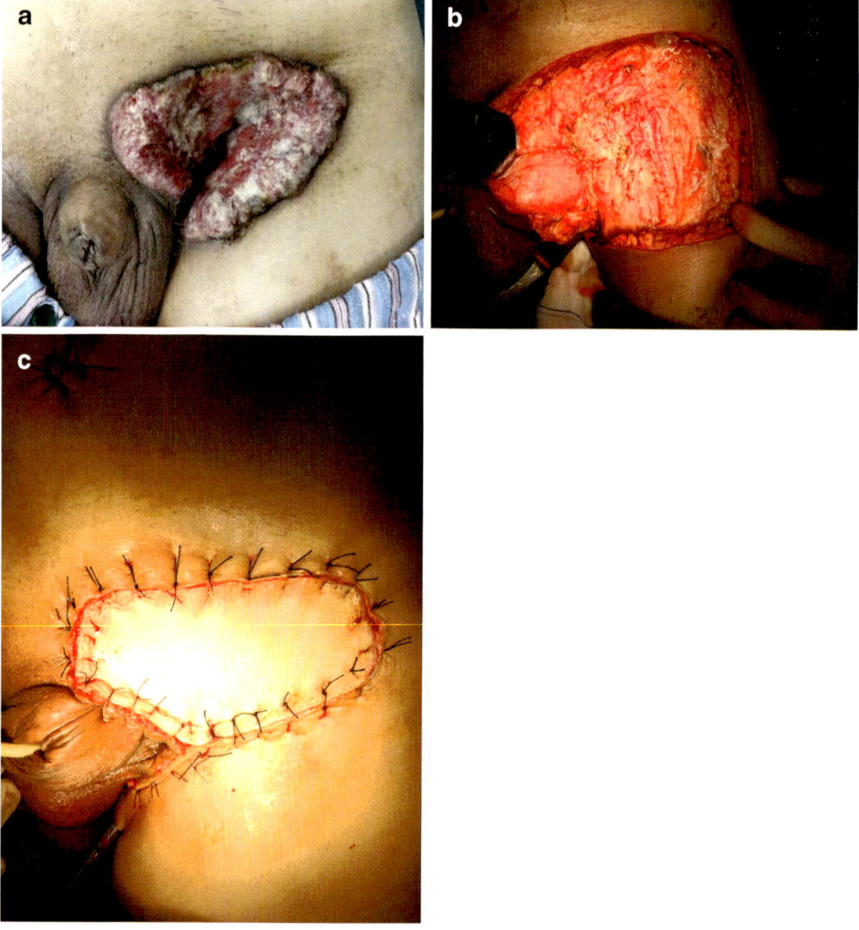

Fig. 7.3 Case 2 Primary closure of the defect using VRAM flaps (**a**) Widespread invasion of the abdominal and groin skin (**b**) Complete removal of tumours (**c**) Closure of the abdominal and groin wound

have symptomatic benefit, alleviating symptoms such as pain and bleeding. It may additionally prevent secondary complications including serious infection and reducing the risk of femoral vessel haemorrhage due to malignant infiltration. Several pedicled flaps have been described for reconstruction following extensive groin dissections. These include the rectus femoris pedicled flap, vertical rectus abdominis myocutaneous (VRAM), anterolateral thigh (ALT), and tensor fascia lata (TFL) flaps. Of these, the VRAM, TFL, and ALT flap have been used most extensively [14].

Pelvic Lymphadenectomy

In general, 20–30% of patients with positive inguinal nodes have positive pelvic nodes [15]. Pelvic lymphadenectomy can be curative in some of these patients, especially those with occult pelvic metastases. Pelvic nodal metastasis are related to the number of positive inguinal metastatic nodes and the presence of extranodal extension.

Indications for Pelvic Lymphadenectomy

In patients with two or more inguinal nodes involved on one side, or if extranodal extension is present, an ipsilateral pelvic lymphadenectomy of the affected side is recommended to be performed in current EAU guidelines.

Boundaries of a Pelvic Node Dissection

Pelvic lymphadenectomy may be performed simultaneously with inguinal lymphadenectomy or as a secondary procedure. If bilateral pelvic lymphadenectomy is indicated this may be performed through a midline suprapubic/extraperitoneal incision.

The boundaries for pelvic node dissection include *Cranially*: the common iliac artery, *caudally*: the inguinal canal, *medially*: the bladder, prostate, and the medial branches of the internal iliac artery, *laterally*: the ilioinguinal nerve and *inferiorly*: the obturator fossa.

Patients with preoperative evidence of pelvic metastases are unlikely to be cured by surgery alone meaning patients are therefore recommended to undergo neoadjuvant chemotherapy. However, even with multimodal treatment, previous studies have shown poor prognosis of patients with pelvic nodal involvement, with 5-year survival rates from 0 to 20% [16].

Key Points

- Penile amputation remains the standard therapy for patients with advanced penile cancer
- Patients with locally advanced penile cancer are at an increased risk for disease-related mortality with surgical treatment alone and are best treated using multimodal approaches.
- Large ulcerating metastatic lymph nodes can be resected surgically as a palliative procedure in those with a good performance status to improve quality of life. Multimodal treatment is however of benefit to these patients.

Revision Questions

Multiple Choice Questions

Case 1

A 52-year-old male presents with fever and dysuria. There is no obvious cause for the fever of 38 °C, without cough, nausea, vomiting or abdominal discomfort. On further questioning the patient complains of dysuria and a weak stream of urine. The patient additionally has a new glans mass which has been worsening for 6 months and has recently become ulcerated in the last 2 weeks.

1. Which investigations should be arranged next?
   A. Pelvic MRI
   B. Chest CT
   C. PET/CT
   D. Blood examination
   E. Biopsy

Case 1 Continued

After receiving 1 week of antibiotics, the patient received a penile biopsy which confirmed the diagnosis of a squamous cell carcinoma. MR subsequently shows a tumour of the glans which is infiltrating into the distal corporal tips.

2. What treatment would you choose for the patient?
   A. Glansectomy
   B. Partial penectomy
   C. Total penectomy
   D. Circumcision
   E. Radiotherapy

Case 2

A 74-year-old male presents with a left inguinal mass for 1 week. Three months ago, the patient underwent a partial penectomy with the postoperative pathology having demonstrated an invasive high grade squamous cell carcinoma. The staging was T1bN0M0. One week ago, the patient found a left large and fixed inguinal mass. He does not have fever, pain. A subsequent fine needle aspiration confirmed metastasis from his penile cancer.

3. What treatment would you choose for the patient?
   A. Anti-infective treatment
   B. Instant Inguinal Lymph Node Dissection
   C. Neoadjuvant chemotherapy
   D. Radiotherapy
   E. palliative chemotherapy

Case 2 Continued

The patient subsequently went on to receive a two-cycle TIP (paclitaxel, ifosfamide and cisplatin) chemotherapy. MR subsequently showed the metastatic lymph node reduced in size remarkably. The treatment effect evaluation was PR.

4. What treatment would you choose next for the patient?
   A. chemotherapy
   B. radiotherapy
   C. Unilateral ILND
   D. bilateral ILND

Case 2 Continued

The patient therefore underwent bilateral ILND. Microscopically, two metastatic inguinal nodes with extranodal extension were found in the left inguinal adipose tissue.

5. What treatment would you choose for the patient next?
   A. adjuvant chemotherapy
   B. adjuvant radiotherapy
   C. one-side pelvic LND
   D. bilateral pelvic LND

Answers

Multiple Choice Questions

1. **A,C,D,E**. The patient had glans mass with infection. The initial diagnosis is penile cancer. Pathological diagnosis is the gold standard of the tumour diagnosis. Pelvic MRI can help to find metastatic lymph node. Blood examination and urinalysis can help to diagnosis of infection, which indicated the rational use of antibiotics.
2. **B**. MRI is showing the tumour to have infiltrated the distal corporal. The first choice for a stage T2–3 penile cancer is partial penectomy. The aim of the surgery is to ensure the tumour-free margins. If the patient is reluctant to do surgery, radiotherapy may be a surrogate treatment.

3. **C**. The patient presented a large a fixed inguinal metastatic lymph node. Thus, the current tumour stage is T1bN3. The patient should undergo comprehensive imaging exanimation to exclude distant metastasis. According to the clinical guidelines, neoadjuvant chemotherapy is the first choice for these patients.
4. **D**. Although the patient had good response to neoadjuvant chemotherapy, an effective operation remains the main methods to cure penile cancer. The primary the tumour was staged as pT1b, bilateral ILND is therefore recommended for the patient.
5. **C**. Overall, 20–30% of patients with positive inguinal nodes have positive pelvic nodes. The patient had two inguinal nodes involved with extranodal extension, an ipsilateral pelvic lymphadenectomy of the affected side is therefore recommended.

Test your learning and check your understanding of this book's contents: use the "Springer Nature Flashcards" app to access questions using ▸ https://sn.pub/1r7Om8. To use the app, please follow the instructions in chapter 1.

References

1. Djajadiningrat RS, Graafland NM, van Werkhoven E, Meinhardt W, Bex A, van der Poel HG, et al. Contemporary management of regional nodes in penile cancer-improvement of survival? J Urol. 2014;191(1):68–73.
2. Solsona E, Iborra I, Ricos JV, Monros JL, Dumont R, Casanova J, et al. Corpus cavernosum invasion and tumor grade in the prediction of lymph node condition in penile carcinoma. Eur Urol. 1992;22(2):115–8.
3. Ficarra V, Akduman B, Bouchot O, Palou J, Tobias-Machado M. Prognostic factors in penile cancer. Urology. 2010;76(2 Suppl 1):S66-73.
4. Velazquez EF, Ayala G, Liu H, Chaux A, Zanotti M, Torres J, et al. Histologic grade and perineural invasion are more important than tumor thickness as predictor of nodal metastasis in penile squamous cell carcinoma invading 5 to 10 mm. Am J Surg Pathol. 2008;32(7):974–9.
5. Minhas S, Kayes O, Hegarty P, Kumar P, Freeman A, Ralph D. What surgical resection margins are required to achieve oncological control in men with primary penile cancer? BJU Int. 2005;96(7):1040–3.
6. Kranz J, Parnham A, Albersen M, Sahdev V, Ziada M, Nigam R, et al. Urethral centralization and pseudo-glans formation after partial penectomy. Urologe A. 2017;56(10):1293–7.
7. de Vries HM, Chipollini J, Slongo J, Boyd F, Korkes F, Albersen M, et al. Outcomes of perineal urethrostomy for penile cancer: a 20-year international multicenter experience. Urol Oncol. 2021;39(8):500. e9- e13
8. Hakenberg OW, Comperat EM, Minhas S, Necchi A, Protzel C, Watkin N. EAU guidelines on penile cancer: 2014 update. Eur Urol. 2015;67(1):142–50.
9. Clark PE, Spiess PE, Agarwal N, Biagioli MC, Eisenberger MA, Greenberg RE, et al. Penile cancer: clinical practice guidelines in oncology. J Natl Compr Cancer Netw. 2013;11(5):594–615.
10. Pagliaro LC, Williams DL, Daliani D, Williams MB, Osai W, Kincaid M, et al. Neoadjuvant paclitaxel, ifosfamide, and cisplatin chemotherapy for metastatic penile cancer: a phase II study. J Clin Oncol. 2010;28(24):3851–7.
11. Shukla CJ, Shabbir M, Feneley MR, Withey S, Muneer A, Minhas S. Palliation of male genital cancers. Clin Oncol (R Coll Radiol). 2010;22(9):747–54.

12. Ottenhof SR, Leone A, Djajadiningrat RS, Azizi M, Zargar K, Kidd LC, et al. Surgical and oncological outcomes in patients after vascularised flap reconstruction for locoregionally advanced penile cancer. Eur Urol Focus. 2019;5(5):867–74.
13. Koifman L, Hampl D, Ginsberg M, Castro RB, Koifman N, Ornellas P, et al. The role of primary inguinal surgical debulking for locally advanced penile cancer followed by reconstruction with myocutaneous flap. Int Braz J Urol. 2021;47(6):1162–75.
14. Alnajjar HM, MacAskill F, Christodoulidou M, Mosahebi A, Akers C, Nigam R, et al. Long-term outcomes for penile cancer patients presenting with advanced N3 disease requiring a myocutaneous flap reconstruction or primary closure-a retrospective single Centre study. Transl Androl Urol. 2019;8(Suppl 1):S13–21.
15. Zhu Y, Zhang SL, Ye DW, Yao XD, Dai B, Zhang HL, et al. Prospectively packaged ilioinguinal lymphadenectomy for penile cancer: the disseminative pattern of lymph node metastasis. J Urol. 2009;181(5):2103–8.
16. Graafland NM, van Boven HH, van Werkhoven E, Moonen LM, Horenblas S. Prognostic significance of extranodal extension in patients with pathological node positive penile carcinoma. J Urol. 2010;184(4):1347–53.

How to Manage the Lymph Nodes in Penile Cancer

8

Giuseppe Fallara, Andrea Salonia, and Asif Muneer

Learning Objectives

After reading this chapter you will be able to:

- Recognise the importance of lymph node staging and management in penile cancer
- Describe commonly utilised nodal staging systems
- Discuss staging methods for evaluating nodal metastasis in patients with penile cancer
- Summarise different surgical and non-surgical treatment methods for patients with nodal metastasis and the common complications of these.

G. Fallara
Division of Experimental Oncology/Unit of Urology, URI, IRCCS Ospedale San Raffaele, Milan, Italy

University Vita-Salute San Raffaele, Milan, Italy

Department of Urology, University College London Hospitals, London, UK

A. Salonia
Division of Experimental Oncology/Unit of Urology, URI, IRCCS Ospedale San Raffaele, Milan, Italy

University Vita-Salute San Raffaele, Milan, Italy

A. Muneer (✉)
Department of Urology, University College London Hospitals, London, UK

National Institute for Health Research (NIHR) Biomedical Research Centre, University College London Hospitals, London, UK

Division of Surgery and Interventional Science, University College London, London, UK

Male Genital Cancer Centre, University College London, London, UK
e-mail: asif.muneer@nhs.net

O. Brunckhorst et al. (eds.), *Penile Cancer – A Practical Guide*, Management of Urology, https://doi.org/10.1007/978-3-031-32681-3_8

Why Lymph Node Dissection Is Important in Penile Cancer

Penile cancer is characterized by early dissemination to the regional lymph nodes; hence, surgical resection of the inguinal lymph nodes is required for staging and treatment of patients with penile cancer [1–3]. Patients with clinically impalpable nodes (cN0) may still have underlying micrometastatic disease. The literature estimates that 0–50% of patients with pT1 disease have lymph node invasion, increasing to 40–100% in those with ≥pT2 disease [4–6].

At presentation, enlarged and palpable lymph nodes are clinically evident in 30–65% of patients; however, metastatic disease is found in almost 45–85% of these cases [7, 8]. In the remaining cases, inflammation/infection in the primary tumour is the main cause of lymphadenopathy. In patients with inguinal lymph node metastases, concomitant metastases to pelvic lymph nodes are present in 22-56% of cases [3, 7]. In a large European study, the risk of inguinal lymph node metastasis was 9% for T1G1/2 cN0 tumours [9], whereas the risk was up to 23% for T1G3 or > T1 cN0 tumours [10], and overall occult micro metastases can be present in 12–24% of patients with penile cancer and impalpable lymph nodes [11].

In the absence of accurate nomograms for prediction of inguinal lymph node involvement, additional risk factors for nodal metastases have been suggested, such as histologic grade (high grade G3 tumours) [6, 12–15], sarcomatoid subtype, lymphatic and venous embolization of the primary tumour [6, 16], perineural invasion [12, 14, 17], growth pattern (endophytic vs exophytic) and increased depth of invasion [18–21], younger age at presentation [15, 22], and some molecular biomarkers such as overexpression of p53 [22–25], SOD2 [18, 26], Ki-67 [24, 27–29], ID1 [30, 31], diffuse PD-L1 expression [24, 32, 33], neutrophil-to-lymphocyte ratios [6, 24, 34], squamous cell carcinoma antigen (SCC-Ag) [6, 24] and serum CRP >20 [30].

The importance of lymph node dissection is not only for the correct staging, and thus for optimized patient counselling and peri-operative multimodal management with neo-adjuvant and adjuvant chemotherapy [3], but also for improved survival [1, 35]. Lymph node invasion has been shown to be the most important prognostic factor for men with penile cancer [6, 7]. In the case of less than 2 unilateral inguinal lymph nodes with metastatic disease, the 5-year overall survival is 80%, being 10–20% in the case of bilateral or pelvic lymph node involvement and less than 10% in the case of extra-nodal extension [3, 36]. Similarly, the 5-year cancer specific survival (CSS) is 85–100%, 79–89%, 17–60% and 0–17%, in the case of pN0, pN1, pN2 and pN3 disease, respectively [6]. However, given the morbidity associated with inguinal lymphadenectomy, the adoption rates of early inguinal lymphadenectomy are low [37–39].

Penile cancer displays a predictable stepwise lymphatic dissemination from the penis to the inguinal lymph nodes first, unilaterally, or bilaterally, followed by drainage to the ipsilateral pelvic lymph nodes [3]. Distant metastases are rare and usually occur only after inguinal and pelvic node involvement [3].

Staging of Lymph Nodes in Penile Cancer

Lymph node staging is based on the tumour–node–metastasis (TNM) classification which was updated in 2018 [40]. Clinical staging is slightly different from pathological staging:

Clinical node staging:

- cN0: no clinically evident nodes
- cN1: palpable mobile unilateral node
- cN2: ≥2 palpable mobile unilateral nodes or bilateral nodes
- cN3: unilateral or bilateral palpable fixed nodal mass or pelvic lymphadenopathy

Pathologic node staging:

- pN0: no lymph node metastasis
- pN1: ≤2 unilateral lymph node metastases, no extranodal extension
- pN2: ≥3 unilateral lymph node metastases or bilateral lymph node metastases, no extranodal extension
- pN3: extranodal extension or pelvic lymph node metastases.

Assessment of Lymph Node Invasion in Penile Cancer

Combined with a clinical examination, cross-sectional imaging for staging is routine and can identify abnormal inguinal or pelvic lymph nodes. Clinical examination of patients with a high body mass index can result in high rates of false negatives due to morphological reasons, as well as micrometastases which can be found in 10–25% of patients with impalpable lymph nodes [9–11, 41, 42]. In addition, in cases of palpable lymph nodes, cross-sectional imaging might help in studying the relationship to adjacent structures. Therefore, imaging before treatment should be included in the diagnostic workup of patients with penile cancer [43]. According to the European Association of Urology 2020 guidelines for penile cancer, if lymph nodes are impalpable, invasive lymph node staging should be offered only to intermediate- and high-risk patients. However, if the inguinal nodes are palpable, staging should include pelvic computed tomography (CT), combined with positron emission tomography (PET), if uncertainty remains [44]. Similarly, according to the National Comprehensive Cancer Network (NCCN) penile cancer guidelines v.2.2022, imaging should be performed in patients with intermediate or high-risk penile cancer and impalpable lymph nodes and in all men with palpable lymph nodes on physical examination. These suggest using either contrast enhanced CT or magnetic resonance imaging (MRI) of the abdomen and pelvis [45]. In the case of bulky inguinal or enlarged pelvic nodes, percutaneous lymph nodes biopsy is suggested [45].

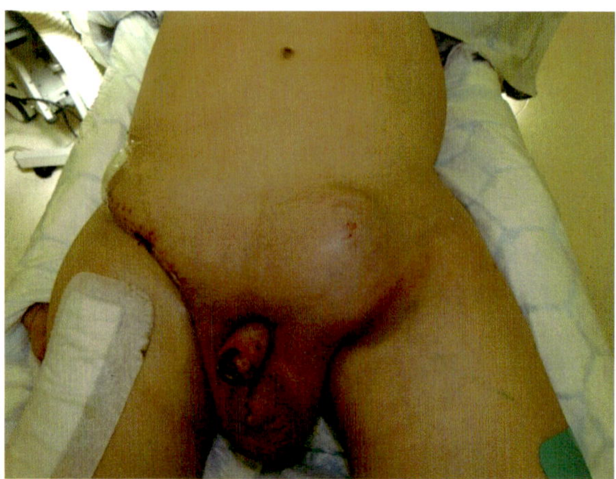

Fig. 8.1 Left bulging mass after glansectomy and right radical inguinal lymph node dissection for cT2N2M0 penile cancer on the glans. The inguinal mass was mobile, dull, not painful. Left radical inguinal lymph node dissection was performed which confirmed the presence of nodal metastasis of penile cancer

Clinical Examination

Clinical evaluation of the groin is an essential step for staging of patients with penile cancer and should aim to assess the presence of palpable lymph nodes, how many are palpable, unilateral or bilateral localization, size, mobility or fixation, the presence of cutaneous erythema, ulcerations or fungating lesions and the relationship to other structures, in particular the femoral vessels (Fig. 8.1).

Inguinal Ultrasonography (US)

The primary role of US in the work-up of patients with penile cancer is to evaluate the groin for morphologically abnormal lymph nodes. A linear probe with high frequencies (7.5 MHz) is usually used to detect enlarged nodes. Morphological changes on ultrasound suggesting metastatic disease include a high longitudinal/transverse diameter ratio and the absence of the lymph node hilum. Sensitivity and specificity of ultrasonography are low; however, accuracy can be improved by using fine needle aspiration (FNA) cytology, with a sensitivity of 39% and a specificity of 90% in the case of enlarged nodes on US scan, and a sensitivity of 93% and a specificity of 91% in the case of palpable nodes [46, 47]. In addition, penile biopsy can be avoided in in the presence of FNA confirmed cytology from palpable inguinal lymph nodes, as the presence of squamous cell carcinoma in the cytology confirms the diagnosis [3].

Cross Sectional Imaging—Computed Tomography (CT) Imaging, Magnetic Resonance Imaging (MRI) and Positron Emission Tomography (PET)/CT

Pelvic CT, MRI and PET/CT are used for pre-operative staging. However, the presence of micrometastases can be underestimated, given their limited spatial resolution (2 mm) [48]. Cross-sectional imaging is used to assess size, location, presence of central necrosis, and the relationship with proximal structures, as well as to evaluate pelvic lymph nodes and distant metastases. NCCN guidelines suggest the use of MRI to aid physical examination in patients where inguinal lymph nodes are difficult to assess [49–51], while the use of 18- fluorodeoxyglucose (FDG) PET/CT is suggested in cN+ cases, especially when more extensive metastatic disease is suspected [52, 53].

Contrast enhanced CT alone has a sensitivity of almost 87% and a specificity of almost 81% when a cut-off of 8 mm is used to identify potentially metastatic lymph nodes [48]. Gadolinum contrast enhanced MRI is likely overlapped with contrast enhanced CT scans for inguinal lymph node staging, however, may provide additional information on primary tumour staging [54]. Accuracy of MRI is similar to CT for inguinal lymph node staging [54]. A systematic review showed a pooled sensitivity of 96% and specificity of 92% for 18F-FDG PET/CT for patients with palpable lymph nodes but 57% for cN0 patients [55]. The association of FNA cytology is believed to increase the sensitivity to 91% and specificity to almost 100% [54]. Finally, in a small cohort study, diagnostic accuracy of 18F-FDG PET/CT for pelvic lymph node staging and distant metastases in cN+ patients has been found to be higher than contrast-enhanced CT alone [56].

Lymph Node Management in Penile Cancer

Indications for Lymph Node Dissection

The presence of metastatic lymph nodes is a poor prognostic indicator for patients with penile cancer. Surgical staging of the inguinal lymph nodes remains central in penile cancer management because 15–24% of patients with cN0 disease may harbour micrometastases and that the correct identification of reactive or malignant lymphadenopathy is challenging in cN+ patients [7, 8, 11]. However, invasive surgery leads to a non-negligible risk of low and high-grade adverse events. Hence, patients with cN0 disease with risk factors for micro metastasis, such as high pT stage, poorly differentiated tumours and lympho-vascular invasion, are offered a risk-adapted approach involving less-invasive groin staging [44, 45].

According to the NCCN guidelines on penile cancer v2.2022, if inguinal lymph nodes are not palpable and the primary lesion is low grade/stage (i.e. Ta, Tis or T1a) surveillance is recommended. However, in cases of high-risk cases (T1b or higher stage, lympho-vascular invasion, or poorly differentiated high-grade disease) dynamic sentinel node biopsy (DSNB) followed by radical inguinal lymph node dissection (ILND) where positive sentinel node(s) are detected, or direct to a radical or modified ILND, are recommended [45].

For palpable lymph nodes, other factors come into play. Firstly, in the case of one or more unilateral non-bulky mobile inguinal lymph nodes, FNA is recommended and if the results are negative for malignancy, excisional biopsy is recommended, whereas, if FNA results are positive for malignancy, radical ILND is recommended on the side of metastatic disease [45]. Any groin with a positive inguinal lymph node requires a radical ILND on the side of the metastatic disease.

Where there is extensive lymph node involvement or extracapsular extension, an ipsilateral pelvic lymphadenectomy (PLND) is recommended [45]. If lymph nodes are bilateral or fixed and results of FNA are positive for malignancy, neoadjuvant chemotherapy followed by ILND and PLND in responders is an option provided that the inguinal lymph nodes are not imminently fungating [45]. Those who are not eligible for neoadjuvant chemotherapy proceed directly to ILND and PLND [45]. Radiation therapy (RT) and chemoradiotherapy are options for patients unfit or unwilling to undergo surgery.

Finally, in the case of bulky lymph nodes with FNA and excisional biopsy negative for metastatic disease, surveillance is recommended although this is a rare occurrence [45]. The EAU guidelines on penile cancer provide similar recommendations, suggesting surveillance for low risk cN0 cases; bilateral modified ILND or DSNB followed by radical or modified ILND on the side of the metastatic disease if sentinel node(s) is positive for malignancy, in case of high risk cN0; bilateral radical ILND in case of cN1/cN2 cases; and neoadjuvant chemotherapy followed by radical ILND in case of cN3 cases [44]. PLDN is recommended in case of pN2 or pN3 disease followed by adjuvant chemotherapy [44].

Dynamic Sentinel Node Biopsy (DSNB)

The stepwise lymphatic drainage from the penis and the subsequent possibility of performing sentinel lymph node (SLN) removal was first demonstrated in 1977 by Cabanas with the use of lymphangiograms [57]. Since then, the technique has evolved and in high volume centres has become the standard of care for surgical staging of the groins for non-palpable lymph nodes. DSNB uses a preoperative peritumoral injection of both ^{99m}Technectium-labelled nanocolloid and a dye, such as patent blue [58, 59]. A single-photon emission CT (SPECT)/CT is used to identify the location of the sentinel node [60, 61]. In practice, one day or up to 4 h before sentinel node surgery 0.3–0.4 mL of ^{99m}Technectium-labelled nanocolloid is injected close to the tumour or proximal to the resection site and conventional planar lymphoscintigraphic images are obtained from all patients. Immediate dynamic (up to 10–20 min) and static imaging at 30 min and 2 h post-injection are obtained [54]. SPECT-CT imaging is performed immediately after the 2-h planar images [60, 61]. Of note, there may be multiple sentinel lymph nodes, and in 80–90% drainage is bilateral [62]. Following the injection all sentinel nodes identified intraoperatively with the preoperative lymphoscintigraphic and SPECT-CT images, and those containing dye, gamma radiation (a gamma ray detection probe is used intraoperatively for this) or both, are removed and sent for pathological assessment [60, 61] (Fig. 8.2). Frozen section analysis of the sentinel lymph node may have a role to indicate for a wider inguinal lymph node dissection in the same surgical session of DSNB, however surgical time and the need to manipulate radioactive specimen should be considered.

Alternatively, to improve diagnostic accuracy of metastatic sentinel node(s), the use of a hybrid fluorescent and radioactive tracer, such as Indocyanine Green–99mTc-nanocolloid, has been proposed (up to a 39% higher detection rate) [63, 64]. The steps are the same, apart from ^{99m}Technectium-labelled nanocolloid is replaced with a hybrid Indocyanine Green–99mTc-nanocolloid is injected before lymphoscintigraphy/SPECT-TC. Here, a fluorescence camera is used for node identification. Perioperative complications rates remain low [63].

To further improve the diagnostic accuracy of the lymph node staging, preoperative inguinal ultrasonography and FNA cytology of morphologically abnormal lymph nodes is performed, reducing the false negative rate to 5% [65, 66]. In addition, intraoperative palpation of nodes, serial sectioning at pathology with intervals at 2 mm of the specimen, immunostaining, repeating DSNB and combination with PET/CT of the specimen might increase the detection of micrometastasis [67–73].

In a large prospective multicentre cohort of more than 600 patients with cN0 disease, a sensitivity of 93%, specificity of 100% and complication rate < 5% has been found using DSNB in high-volume centres, figures that were confirmed by several other retrospective studies [58, 62, 74, 75]. However, concerns of a high false-negative and complication rates in non-centralized health-care systems and in those with poor access to nuclear medicine, along with a steep learning curve, have somewhat hindered the use of DSNB [76].

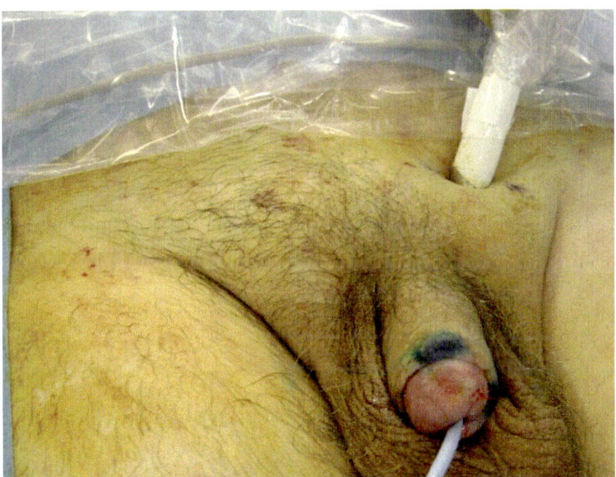

Fig. 8.2 Example of left dynamic sentinel node biopsy, after wide local excision of penile cancer of the glans (cT1N0M0). The 99mTechnectium-labelled nanocolloid radiotracer is injected in the morning and lymphoscintigraphic images are taken at 0, 10, 20 and 30 min after injection while a SPECT-CT is performed 2 h after the injection. Patent blue dye is injected just before surgery. During surgery a gamma probe, together with palpation and direct visualisation of the patent blue dye, are used to identify the sentinel lymph node(s)

Inguinal Lymph Node Dissection (ILND)

ILND remains the standard of care in the clinical staging of patients with penile cancer [44, 45]. The extent of the lymph node dissection should be adapted to the clinical stage. For patients without palpable lymph nodes (cN0), DSNB or where this is not available then superficial ILND is recommended, which is associated with a reduced complication rate compared to radical ILND [44, 45]. On the other hand, all patients with histologically proven lymph node metastases after DSNB or FNA and/or with palpable large node(s) should undergo a radical ILND on the same side of the metastatic disease [44, 45]. There is limited literature reporting on the ideal number of lymph nodes to be removed at ILND, but it has been suggested that the removal of more than 15 nodes is associated with better survival outcomes [77].

Radical ILND involves the removal of the superficial and deep inguinal lymph nodes, which are separated by the fascia lata in the femoral triangle. The boundaries of the dissection consist superiorly of the inguinal ligament, medially of the adductor longus muscle, and laterally of the medial border of the sartorius muscle while the floor for the superficial dissection consists of the fascia lata and for the deep dissection of the pectineus muscle. Radical ILND is associated with a non-negligible rate of short and long terms complications, with overall complication rates up to 50–60% and severe complication (Clavien Dindo ≥3) rates up to 10% of cases [78]. Wound infection has been reported in up to 43% of cases; up to 24% of cases will develop a seroma; it has been reported a 5-7% incidence of deep venous thrombosis or pulmonary embolism; rates of lymphocele and lymphedema to the lower limb and scrotum ranged between 9–16% and 16–50%, respectively (Fig. 8.3) [79]. Such a scenario leads to a reduction in the quality of life for these patients [80].

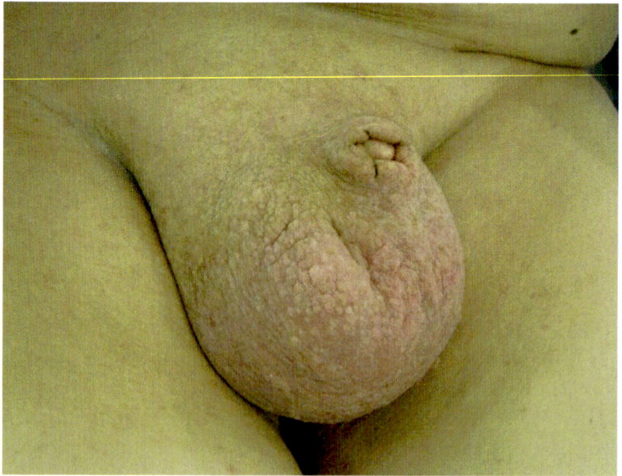

Fig. 8.3 Lymphoedema of the scrotum is a possible complication of ILND with an incidence of 50-60% of cases. Surgical indications are mainly for patient discomfort, and bulky lymphoedema

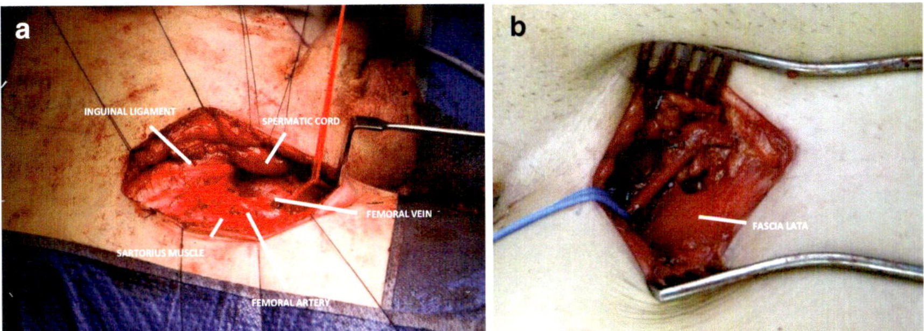

Fig. 8.4 (**a**) Example of radical inguinal lymph node dissection. Skin incision is performed almost 2 cm below the inguinal ligament and dissection is conducted above and below the fascia lata. (**b**) Example of superficial inguinal lymph node dissection. Skin incision is always performed almost 2 cm below the inguinal ligament, shorter than in the case of radical ILND, and dissection is performed above the fascia lata

Various techniques have been described to reduce the morbidity related to radical ILND:

- The use of superficial ILND alone, in cN0 cases. The superficial inguinal nodes are those found above the fascia lata. These nodes are evaluated intra-operatively using frozen section analysis and, if positive, the surgery proceeds to a radical ILND [44, 45].
- The use of modified ILND, in cN0 cases. The modified ILND, was first described by Catalona et al. in 1988 and reduces the dissection area with a smaller skin incision [81]. Laterally dissection should not go beyond the lateral border of the femoral artery and caudally dissection not beyond the fossa ovalis. Additionally, the Scarpa's fascia and the saphenous vein are preserved, and no sartorius muscle transposition is performed. The nodes are evaluated intra-operatively using frozen section and, if positive for malignancy, dissection of the deep inguinal nodes is performed [81, 82]. Modified ILND has been shown to reduce complications related to lymphatic drainage to 10–36%, likely thanks to the preservation of the saphenous vein (Fig. 8.4) [81, 83].
- Laparoscopic and robot-assisted ILND have also been adopted to reduce complications by making smaller skin incisions [84–87]. Despite initial promising results, the lack of solid data from randomized control trials (difficult to design owing to the rarity of penile cancer), the fact that only small case series have been published and the likely long learning curve, hindered its spread.

Pelvic Lymph Node Dissection (PLND)

In patients with penile cancer with two or more positive inguinal lymph nodes (pN2) or extranodal extension (pN3), an ipsilateral PLND is indicated. Ipsilateral

PLND is recommended since cross-over of metastatic disease from the contralateral groin has not been reported [44, 45]. PLND can be performed during the same operative setting of ILND or in a delayed fashion. Up to 23% of cases with two positive inguinal lymph nodes and 56% of cases with three positive inguinal lymph nodes or extranodal extension harbors metastatic pelvic lymph nodes [41]. The 5-year CSS of patients with pelvic nodal metastasis is worse compared to that of patients with only inguinal node metastasis, 71% vs 33.2%, respectively [44, 88]. PLND can be performed via an open, laparoscopic or robot-assisted surgery. During PLND, nodes are excised around the obturator and external iliac regions.

Radiotherapy

Primary radiotherapy to inguinal/pelvic lymph nodes in cases of anal, vulvar or cervical squamous cell carcinomas has a primary role, suggesting a potential application also in lymph node metastases from penile cancer. However, there are few published data on the effect of radiotherapy in this setting and a systematic review failed to demonstrate any benefit of adjuvant inguinal radiotherapy following ILND [89–92]. As such, while the NCCN guidelines suggest radiotherapy as an option among definitive treatments (especially for patients unfit for surgery), the EAU guidelines only recommend it for palliation [44, 45].

Neoadjuvant and Adjuvant Chemotherapy

As previously outlined, patients with penile cancer and multiple inguinal and pelvic lymph node metastases, have a poor prognosis. Current guidelines suggest the use of neoadjuvant therapy before lymphadenectomy in patients with locally advanced disease, i.e. fixed or bulky inguinal lymph nodes or pelvic lymph node involvement (cN3), based on a combination of taxanes and cisplatin (TIP – paclitaxel, ifosfamide and cisplatin) [44, 45, 93, 94]. Overall, the pathological complete response rate in a large multicentre retrospective analysis reached 13%, the clinical objective response rate almost 50%, although the 2-year overall survival remained suboptimal (35.8%) [95, 96].

In addition, adjuvant therapy with a combination of cisplatin and taxanes (TIP) or 5-fluorouracil and cisplatin has been suggested in highly selected case, i.e. patients with pelvic lymph node metastases, extranodal extension, ≥4 cm tumor in the lymph node or bilateral inguinal involvement [44, 45, 97, 98]. Reports of survival outcomes are scarce and indicate a poor 5-year overall survival, around 50% [95, 99, 100]. Evidence on systemic therapy in this setting is scarce, restricting therapeutic recommendations. Finally, the use of other systemic treatments (e.g. immunotherapy) is being currently tested in clinical trials and might play a role changing clinical practice in the following years.

Key Points

- A significant reduction in survival is found in patients with penile cancer and inguinal lymph node metastasis
- Penile cancer displays a predictable stepwise lymphatic dissemination from the penis to the inguinal lymph nodes first, unilaterally or bilaterally, followed by drainage to the ipsilateral pelvic lymph nodes
- Clinical examination and imaging with CT, MRI or 18-FDG/CT play a central role in determining the presence of enlarged and/or fixed lymph nodes
- Radical inguinal lymph node dissection remains the gold standard for the management of inguinal lymph nodes in men with high-risk penile cancer and non-palpable lymph nodes and for those with palpable lymph nodes, despite the high rates of complications. Indeed, other techniques have been proposed, such as the use of dynamic sentinel node biopsy, the modified lymph node dissection and the superficial lymph node dissection, which use however should be restricted to cN0 cases
- The use of neo-adjuvant and adjuvant chemotherapy with combination of taxanes/5- fluorouracile and cisplatin has the potential to increase overall survival in c/pN+ patients

Revision Questions

Multiple Choice Questions

1. What is the probability that impalpable inguinal lymph nodes harbour metastatic disease in men with penile cancer?
   A. Almost 0%, that is why no further investigations must be performed in these patients
   B. Between 10–25%, that is why a risk-adopted stepwise approach is taken
   C. Around 60–75%, hence why nearly all patients undergo sampling unless contraindicated
   D. Between 90–100%, which is why every patient with a diagnosis of penile cancer must be submitted to inguinal lymph-node dissection
2. Are MRI, CT or 18-FGD PET/CT recommended for nodal staging in every patient diagnosed with penile cancer and palpable lymph nodes?
   A. Yes, imaging should always be performed
   B. No, imaging should only be performed in selected cN+ patients
   C. No, given their low diagnostic accuracy they are never performed
3. 65-year-old men was referred with an enlarging lesion on the glans penis. Examination of the genitalia revealed an exophytic lesion extending from the glans and into the distal corpora. The scrotum and testes were normal. The examination of the groins revealed enlarged bilateral inguinal lymph-nodes. Which are the following steps in the diagnostic work-up staging:

   A. No further investigation needed, the patient must undergo a total penectomy and a bilateral radical lymph node dissection
   B. A biopsy of the penis should be performed followed by a total penectomy. The inguinal nodes can be removed by sentinel node biopsy.
   C. FNA cytology from the inguinal nodes is enough to confirm the diagnosis and further staging using CT and penile MRI should be performed.
4. The patient underwent partial penectomy, reconstruction of new urethral meatus and radical inguinal lymphadenectomy bilaterally. The histopathology report confirmed a squamous cell carcinoma of the penis stage pT3N2M0. Which of the following is true regarding the indications for dynamic sentinel lymph node biopsy (DSNB):
   A. DSNB should be performed in every patient with penile cancer
   B. DSNB plays a pivotal role in the staging of men with penile cancer and non-palpable lymph nodes
   C. DSNB is important in staging men with penile cancer and palpable lymph nodes
   D. DSNB only has a marginal role and should be performed in the setting of clinical trials
5. A 53-year-old patient comes to your clinic with a slightly ulcerated mass on his glans which does not occlude the urethral meatus. Multiple bilateral inguinal lymph-nodes are palpable with a bigger fixed mass on the left groin. The patient does not have other comorbidities and renal and liver function are normal. The lesion on the glans does not involve the corpora cavernosa on penile MRI. Both the primary and the inguinal nodes bilaterally were positive for at 18-FDG PET/CT and a FNA on the left inguinal node confirmed metastasis of squamous cell carcinoma. The tumor is then staged as cT1N3M0. The following steps according to the EAU guidelines 2021 on penile cancer should be:
   A. Neoadjuvant chemotherapy with four cycles of TIP, subsequent re-staging with imaging and surgery (glansecotmy + bilateral radical ILND)
   B. Surgery (glansecotmy for the primary and bilateral radical ILND) should not be delayed since evidence on NAC efficacy is poor

Answers

Multiple Choice Questions

1. **B.** In fact, despite clinical examination and diagnostic work-up might show no evidence of metastatic disease still up to 25% of cases harbours micro-metastasis. Known risk factors for inguinal nodal micrometastasis are advanced tumour stage and grade, growth pattern (endophytic vs exophytic) and increased depth of invasion, lymphatic and venous embolization, perineural invasion, younger patient age at diagnosis and some molecular biomarkers such as overexpression of p53, SOD2, Ki-67, ID1, diffuse PD-L1 expression, neutrophil-to-lymphocyte ratios, squamous cell carcinoma antigen (SCC-Ag) and serum CRP >20.

2. **A.** International guidelines suggest the use of multimodal imaging for staging of men with penile cancer and palpable lymph nodes, with the aim of assessing number, dimension and eventual exteranodal invasion of suspected lymph nodes. FNA can improve sensitivity and specificity of palpable nodal staging.
3. **C.** In light of the hypothesis of a diagnosis of advanced penile cancer, the stage of this patient is cT3N2M0; thus, routine investigations include the study of cancer involvement of the penis, with penile MRI; the inguinal lymph nodes should be studied with US scan and CT/18-FDG PET/CT or MRI and FNA cytology; finally, pelvic and distant metastasis should be investigated with pelvic, abdominal and chest CT imaging. In this case, FNA confirmed the suspicion of squamous cell carcinoma of the penis, and an initial involvement of the corpora cavernosa was found at local staging with MRI. Apart from enlarged inguinal lymph-nodes, no pelvic or distant metastases were found at systemic staging.
4. **B.** In fact, dynamic sentinel node biopsy is recommended by guidelines in the setting of cN0 penile cancer in order to reduce the use of ILND only in case of evidence of metastatic disease at DSNB and to reduce its related complications.
5. **A.** The patient was submitted to four cycles of neoadjuvant therapy with TIP which was well tolerated. A significant response was observed in both the groins and the primary. Subsequently, the patient was submitted to consolidative surgery with a glansectomy and bilateral radical ILND. Final surgical pathology revealed no invasion of the corpora or cavernosa and no residual cancer in the inguinal lymph nodes (AJCC Stage 1: ypT1aN0M0, Grade 2).

Test your learning and check your understanding of this book's contents: use the "Springer Nature Flashcards" app to access questions using ▶ https://sn.pub/1r7Om8. To use the app, please follow the instructions in chapter 1.

References

1. Ornellas AA. Management of penile cancer. J Surg Oncol. 2008;97(3):199–200.
2. Chipollini J, Necchi A, Spiess PE. Outcomes for patients with node-positive penile cancer: impact of perioperative systemic therapies and the importance of surgical intervention. Eur Urol. 2018;74(2):241–2.
3. Thomas A, Necchi A, Muneer A, Tobias-Machado M, Tran ATH, Rompuy A-SV, et al. Penile cancer. Nat Rev Dis Primers. 2021;7(1):11.
4. Villavicencio H, Rubio-Briones J, Regalado R, Chéchile G, Algaba F, Palou J. Grade, local stage and growth pattern as prognostic factors in carcinoma of the penis. Eur Urol. 1997;32(4):442–7.
5. Lopes A, Hidalgo GS, Kowalski LP, Torloni H, Rossi BM, Fonseca FP. Prognostic factors in carcinoma of the penis: multivariate analysis of 145 patients treated with amputation and lymphadenectomy. J Urol. 1996;156(5):1637–42.
6. Ficarra V, Akduman B, Bouchot O, Palou J, Tobias-Machado M. Prognostic factors in penile cancer. Urology. 2010;76(2):S66–73.

7. Djajadiningrat RS, Graafland NM, van Werkhoven E, Meinhardt W, Bex A, van der Poel HG, et al. Contemporary management of regional nodes in penile cancer—improvement of survival? J Urol. 2014;191(1):68–73.
8. Srinivas V, Morse MJ, Herr HW, Sogani PC, Whitmore WF. Penile cancer: relation of extent of nodal metastasis to survival. J Urol. 1987;137(5):880–1.
9. Hughes BE, Leijte JAP, Kroon BK, Shabbir MA, Swallow TW, Heenan SD, et al. Lymph node metastasis in intermediate-risk penile squamous cell cancer: a two-Centre experience. Eur Urol. 2010;57(4):688–92.
10. Graafland NM, Lam W, Leijte JAP, Yap T, Gallee MPW, Corbishley C, et al. Prognostic factors for occult inguinal lymph node involvement in penile carcinoma and assessment of the high-risk EAU subgroup: a two-institution analysis of 342 clinically node-negative patients. Eur Urol. 2010;58(5):742–7.
11. Misra S, Chaturvedi A, Misra NC. Penile carcinoma: a challenge for the developing world. Lancet Oncol. 2004;5(4):240–7.
12. Zekan DS, Dahman A, Hajiran AJ, Luchey AM, Chahoud J, Spiess PE. Prognostic predictors of lymph node metastasis in penile cancer: a systematic review. Int Braz J Urol. 2021;47(5):943–56.
13. Theodorescu D, Russo P, Zhang ZF, Morash C, Fair WR. Outcomes of initial surveillance of invasive squamous cell carcinoma of the penis and negative nodes. J Urol. 1996;155(5):1626–31.
14. Velazquez EF, Ayala G, Liu H, Chaux A, Zanotti M, Torres J, et al. Histologic grade and perineural invasion are more important than tumor thickness as predictor of nodal metastasis in penile squamous cell carcinoma invading 5 to 10 mm. Am J Surg Pathol. 2008;32(7):974–9.
15. Alkatout I, Naumann CM, Hedderich J, Hegele A, Bolenz C, Jünemann K-P, et al. Squamous cell carcinoma of the penis: predicting nodal metastases by histologic grade, pattern of invasion and clinical examination. Urol Oncol. 2011;29(6):774–81.
16. Ficarra V, Maffei N, Piacentini I, Rabi NA, Cerruto MA, Artibani W. Local treatment of penile squamous cell carcinoma. Urol Int. 2002;69(3):169–73.
17. Zhou X, Qi F, Zhou R, Wang S, Wang Y, Wang Y, et al. The role of perineural invasion in penile cancer: a meta-analysis and systematic review. Biosci Rep. 2018;38(5):BSR20180333.
18. Emerson RE, Ulbright TM, Eble JN, Geary WA, Eckert GJ, Cheng L. Predicting cancer progression in patients with penile squamous cell carcinoma: the importance of depth of invasion and vascular invasion. Modern Pathol. 2001;14(10):963–8.
19. Dai B, Ye DW, Kong YY, Yao XD, Zhang HL, Shen YJ. Predicting regional lymph node metastasis in Chinese patients with penile squamous cell carcinoma: the role of histopathological classification, tumor stage and depth of invasion. J Urol. 2006;176(4):1431–5.
20. Zhu Y, Zhou XY, Yao XD, Dai B, Ye DW. The prognostic significance of p53, Ki-67, epithelial cadherin and matrix metalloproteinase-9 in penile squamous cell carcinoma treated with surgery. BJU Int. 2007;100(1):204–8.
21. Pizzocaro G, Piva L, Bandieramonte G, Tanac S. Up-to-date management of carcinoma of the penis. Eur Urol. 1997;32(1):5–15.
22. Qu XM, Siemens DR, Louie AV, Yip D, Mahmud A. Validation of predictors for lymph node status in penile cancer: results from a population-based cohort. Can Urol Assoc J. 2017;12(4):119–25.
23. Lopes A, Bezerra ALR, Pinto CAL, Serrano SV, de Mello CA, Villa LL. p53 as a new prognostic factor for lymph node metastasis in penile carcinoma: analysis of 82 patients treated with amputation and bilateral lymphadenectomy. J Urol. 2002;168(1):81–6.
24. Hu J, Cui Y, Liu P, Zhou X, Ren W, Chen J, et al. Predictors of inguinal lymph node metastasis in penile cancer patients: a meta-analysis of retrospective studies. Cancer Manag Res. 2019;11:6425–41.
25. Li K, Sun J, Wei X, Wu G, Wang F, Fan C, et al. Prognostic value of lymphovascular invasion in patients with squamous cell carcinoma of the penis following surgery. BMC Cancer. 2019;19(1):476.
26. Termini L, Fregnani JH, Boccardo E, da Costa WH, Longatto-Filho A, Andreoli MA, et al. SOD2 immunoexpression predicts lymph node metastasis in penile cancer. Bmc Clin Pathol. 2015;15(1):3.

27. Maciel CVDM, Machado RD, Morini MA, Mattos PAL, dos Reis R, dos Reis RB, et al. External validation of nomogram to predict inguinal lymph node metastasis in patients with penile cancer and clinically negative lymph nodes. Int Braz J Urol. 2019;45(4):671–8.
28. Ramkumar A, Seshadri RA, Narayanaswamy K, Balasubramanian S. Risk factors for lymph node metastasis in clinically node-negative penile cancer patients. Int J Urol. 2009;16(4):383–6.
29. Warli SM, Siregar GP. Over-expression of Ki-67 as a predictor of lymph node metastasis in penile cancer patients. F1000research. 2020;9:289.
30. Ghazal AA, Steffens S, Steinestel J, Lehmann R, Schnoeller TJ, Schulte-Hostede A, et al. Elevated C-reactive protein values predict nodal metastasis in patients with penile cancer. BMC Urol. 2013;13(1):53.
31. Hu X, Chen M, Li Y, Wang Y, Wen S, Jun F. Overexpression of ID1 promotes tumor progression in penile squamous cell carcinoma. Oncol Rep. 2019;41(2):1091–100.
32. Unadkat P, Fleishman A, Olumi AF, Wagner A, Chang P, Kim SP, et al. Contemporary incidence and predictors of occult inguinal lymph node metastases in men with clinically node-negative (cN0) penile cancer. Urology. 2021;153:221–7.
33. Su X, Zhang J, Fu C, Xiao M, Wang C. Recurrent metastatic penile cancer patient with positive PD-L1 expression obtained significant benefit from immunotherapy: a case report and literature review. Oncotargets Ther. 2020;13:3319–24.
34. Azizi M, Peyton CC, Boulware DC, Chipollini J, Juwono T, Pow-Sang JM, et al. Prognostic value of neutrophil-to-lymphocyte ratio in penile squamous cell carcinoma patients undergoing inguinal lymph node dissection. Eur Urol Focus. 2019;5(6):1085–90.
35. Kroon BK, Horenblas S, Lont A, Tanis PJ, Gallee MPW, Nieweg OE. Patients with penile carcinoma benefit from immediate resection of clinically occult lymph node metastases. J Urol. 2005;173(3):816–9.
36. Pagliaro LC, Crook J. Multimodality therapy in penile cancer: when and which treatments? World J Urol. 2009;27(2):221–5.
37. Spiess PE, Izawa JI, Bassett R, Kedar D, Busby JE, Wong F, et al. Preoperative lymphoscintigraphy and dynamic sentinel node biopsy for staging penile cancer: results with pathological correlation. J Urol. 2007;177(6):2157–61.
38. Ross G, Shoaib T, Scott J, Soutar DS, Gray H, Mackie R. The learning curve for sentinel node biopsy in malignant melanoma. Br J Plast Surg. 2002;55(4):298–301.
39. Woldu SL, Ci B, Hutchinson RC, Krabbe L-M, Singla N, Passoni NM, et al. Usage and survival implications of surgical staging of inguinal lymph nodes in intermediate- to high-risk, clinical localized penile cancer: a propensity-score matched analysis. Urol Oncol. 2018;36(4):159.e7–159.e17.
40. Amin MB, Edge SB, Greene FL, Byrd DR, Brookland RK, Washington MK, et al., editors. AJCC cancer staging manual [Internet]. Vol. XVII. Springer International Publishing; 2017 [cited 2017]. 1032 p. Available from: https://link.springer.com/gp/book/9783319406176
41. Leone A, Diorio GJ, Pettaway C, Master V, Spiess PE. Contemporary management of patients with penile cancer and lymph node metastasis. Nat Rev Urol. 2017;14(6):335–47.
42. Derakhshani P, Neubauer S, Braun M, Bargmann H, Heidenreich A, Engelmann U. Results and 10-year follow-up in patients with squamous cell carcinoma of the penis. Urol Int. 1999;62(4):238–44.
43. Heyns CF, Fleshner N, Sangar V, Schlenker B, Yuvaraja TB, van Poppel H. Management of the lymph nodes in penile cancer. Urology. 2010;76(2):S43–57.
44. Hakenberg OW, Compérat E, Minhas S, Necchi A, Protzel C, Watkin N, et al. EAU Guidelines on Penile Cancer 2020. In: Office EG, editor. 2020 [cited 2022 Feb 5]. Available from: https://uroweb.org/wp-content/uploads/EAU-Guidelines-on-Penile-Cancer-2020.pdf
45. (NCCN) NCCN, editor. NCCN Clinical Practice Guidelines in Oncology. Penile Cancer. Version 2.2022. In 2022 [cited 2022 Feb 5]. Available from: https://www.nccn.org/professionals/physician_gls/pdf/penile.pdf
46. Ornellas AA, Nóbrega BLB, Chin EWK, Wisnescky A, da Silva PCB, Schwindt ABDS. Prognostic factors in invasive squamous cell carcinoma of the penis: analysis of 196 patients treated at the Brazilian National Cancer Institute. J Urol. 2008;180(4):1354–9.

47. Kirrander P, Sherif A, Friedrich B, Lambe M, Håkansson U, Register SC of the SNPC. Swedish National Penile Cancer Register: incidence, tumour characteristics, management and survival. BJU Int. 2016;117(2):287–92.
48. Graafland NM, Teertstra HJ, Besnard APE, van Boven HH, Horenblas S. Identification of high risk pathological node positive penile carcinoma: value of preoperative computerized tomography imaging. J Urol. 2011;185(3):881–7.
49. Mueller-Lisse UG, Scher B, Scherr MK, Seitz M. Functional imaging in penile cancer & colon; PET/computed tomography, MRI, and sentinel lymph node biopsy. Curr Opin Urol. 2008;18(1):105–10.
50. Hedgire SS, Pargaonkar VK, Elmi A, Harisinghani AM, Harisinghani MG. Pelvic nodal imaging. Radiol Clin N Am. 2012;50(6):1111–25.
51. Caso JR, Rodriguez AR, Correa J, Spies PE. Update in the management of penile cancer. Int Braz J Urol. 2009;35(4):406–15.
52. Salazar A, Júnior EP, Salles PGO, Silva-Filho R, Reis EA, Mamede M. 18F-FDG PET/CT as a prognostic factor in penile cancer. Eur J Nucl Med Mol I. 2019;46(4):855–63.
53. Scher B, Seitz M, Albinger W, Reiser M, Schlenker B, Stief C, et al. PET in oncology. Recent Results Canc. 2008:159–79.
54. Bloom JB, Stern M, Patel NH, Zhang M, Phillips JL. Detection of lymph node metastases in penile cancer. Transl Androl Urol. 2018;7(5):879–86.
55. Sadeghi R, Gholami H, Zakavi SR, Kakhki VRD, Horenblas S. Accuracy of 18F-FDG PET/CT for diagnosing inguinal lymph node involvement in penile squamous cell carcinoma. Clin Nucl Med. 2012;37(5):436–41.
56. Ottenhof SR, Vegt E. The role of PET/CT imaging in penile cancer. Transl Androl Urol. 2017;6(5):833–8.
57. Cabanas RM. An approach for the treatment of penile carcinoma. Cancer. 1977;39(2):456–66.
58. Lam W, Alnajjar HM, La-Touche S, Perry M, Sharma D, Corbishley C, et al. Dynamic sentinel lymph node biopsy in patients with invasive squamous cell carcinoma of the penis: a prospective study of the long-term outcome of 500 inguinal basins assessed at a single institution. Eur Urol. 2013;63(4):657–63.
59. Horenblas S, Kroger R, Gallee MPW, Newling DWW, Tinteren HV. Ultrasound in squamous cell carcinoma of the penis; a useful addition to clinical staging? A comparison of ultrasound with histopathology. Urology. 1994;43(5):702–7.
60. Leijte JAP, Olmos RAV, Nieweg OE, Horenblas S. Anatomical mapping of lymphatic drainage in penile carcinoma with SPECT-CT: implications for the extent of inguinal lymph node dissection. Eur Urol. 2008;54(4):885–92.
61. Lützen U, Naumann CM, Marx M, Zhao Y, Jüptner M, Baumann R, et al. A study on the value of computer-assisted assessment for SPECT/CT-scans in sentinel lymph node diagnostics of penile cancer as well as clinical reliability and morbidity of this procedure. Cancer Imaging. 2016;16(1):29.
62. Sadeghi R, Gholami H, Zakavi SR, Kakhki VRD, Tabasi KT, Horenblas S. Accuracy of sentinel lymph node biopsy for inguinal lymph node staging of penile squamous cell carcinoma: systematic review and meta-analysis of the literature. J Urol. 2012;187(1):25–31.
63. Dell'Oglio P, de Vries HM, Mazzone E, KleinJan GH, Donswijk ML, van der Poel HG, et al. Hybrid indocyanine green–99mTc-nanocolloid for single-photon emission computed tomography and combined radio- and fluorescence-guided sentinel node biopsy in penile cancer: results of 740 inguinal basins assessed at a single institution. Eur Urol. 2020;78(6):865–72.
64. Brouwer OR, Buckle T, Vermeeren L, Klop WMC, Balm AJM, van der Poel HG, et al. Comparing the hybrid fluorescent–radioactive tracer indocyanine green–99mTc-Nanocolloid with 99mTc-Nanocolloid for sentinel node identification: a validation study using lymphoscintigraphy and SPECT/CT. J Nucl Med. 2012;53(7):1034–40.
65. Leijte JAP, Kroon BK, Olmos RAV, Nieweg OE, Horenblas S. Reliability and safety of current dynamic sentinel node biopsy for penile carcinoma. Eur Urol. 2007;52(1):170–7.
66. Leijte JAP, van der Ploeg IMC, Olmos RAV, Nieweg OE, Horenblas S. Visualization of tumor blockage and rerouting of lymphatic drainage in penile cancer patients by use of SPECT/CT. J Nucl Med. 2009;50(3):364–7.

67. Kroon BK, Horenblas S, Estourgie SH, Lont AP, Rav O, Nieweg OE. How to avoid false-negative dynamic sentinel node procedures in penile carcinoma. J Urol. 2004;171(6):2191–4.
68. Kroon BK, Horenblas S, Deurloo EE, Nieweg OE, Teertstra HJ. Ultrasonography-guided fine-needle aspiration cytology before sentinel node biopsy in patients with penile carcinoma. BJU Int. 2005;95(4):517–21.
69. Jakobsen JK, Alslev L, Ipsen P, Costa JC, Krarup KP, Sommer P, et al. DaPeCa-3: promising results of sentinel node biopsy combined with 18F-fluorodeoxyglucose positron emission tomography/computed tomography in clinically lymph node-negative patients with penile cancer—a national study from Denmark. BJU Int. 2016;118(1):102–11.
70. Hadway P, Smith Y, Corbishley C, Heenan S, Watkin NA. Evaluation of dynamic lymphoscintigraphy and sentinel lymph-node biopsy for detecting occult metastases in patients with penile squamous cell carcinoma. BJU Int. 2007;100(3):561–5.
71. Crawshaw JW, Hadway P, Hoffland D, Bassingham S, Corbishley CM, Smith Y, et al. Sentinel lymph node biopsy using dynamic lymphoscintigraphy combined with ultrasound-guided fine needle aspiration in penile carcinoma. Br J Radiol. 2009;82(973):41–8.
72. Sahdev V, Albersen M, Christodoulidou M, Parnham A, Malone P, Nigam R, et al. Management of non-visualization following dynamic sentinel lymph node biopsy for squamous cell carcinoma of the penis. BJU Int. 2017;119(4):573–8.
73. Graafland NM, Leijte JAP, Olmos RAV, Boven HHV, Nieweg OE, Horenblas S. Repeat dynamic sentinel node biopsy in locally recurrent penile carcinoma. BJU Int. 2010;105(8):1121–4.
74. Kroon BK, Lont AP, Rav O, Nieweg OE, Horenblas S, Morbidity of dynamic sentinel node biopsy in penile carcinoma. J Urol. 2005;173(3):813–5.
75. Leijte JAP, Hughes B, Graafland NM, Kroon BK, Olmos RAV, Nieweg OE, et al. Two-center evaluation of dynamic sentinel node biopsy for squamous cell carcinoma of the penis. J Clin Oncol. 2009;27(20):3325–9.
76. Nabavizadeh R, Petrinec B, Nabavizadeh B, Singh A, Rawal S, Master V. Inguinal lymph node dissection in the era of minimally invasive surgical technology. Urol Oncol Seminars Orig Investigations. 2020;
77. Soodana-Prakash N, Koru-Sengul T, Miao F, Lopategui DM, Savio LF, Moore KJ, et al. Lymph node yield as a predictor of overall survival following inguinal lymphadenectomy for penile cancer. Urol Oncol. 2018;36(10):471.e19–27.
78. Gupta MK, Patel AP, Master VA. Technical considerations to minimize complications of inguinal lymph node dissection. Transl Androl Urol. 2017;6(5):820–5.
79. Chipollini J, Garcia-Castaneda J, la Rosa AH-D, Cheriyan S, Azizi M, Spiess PE. Important surgical concepts and techniques in inguinal lymph node dissection. Curr Opin Urol. 2019;29(3):286–92.
80. Coba G, Patel T. Penile cancer: managing sexual dysfunction and improving quality of life after therapy. Curr Urol Rep. 2021;22(2):8.
81. Catalona WJ. Modified inguinal lymphadenectomy for carcinoma of the penis with preservation of saphenous veins: technique and preliminary results. J Urol. 1988;140(2):306–10.
82. Selçuk İ, Akdemir HA, Ersak B, Tatar İ, Sargon MF, Güngör T. Inguinofemoral lymphadenectomy and femoral dissection: cadaveric educational video. J Turkish Ger Gynecol Assoc. 2021;22(2):155–7.
83. Niyogi D, Noronha J, Pal M, Bakshi G, Prakash G. Management of clinically node-negative groin in patients with penile cancer. Indian J Urol Iju J Urol Soc India. 2020;36(1):8–15.
84. Hora M, Trávníček I, Nykodýmová Š, Ferda J, Kacerovská D, Michalová K, et al. VEILND (video endoscopic inguinal lymph node dissection) with florescence indocyanine green (ICG): a novel technique to identify the sentinel lymph node in men with ≥pT1G2 and cN0 penile cancer. Contrast Media Mol I. 2021;2021:5575730.
85. Tobias-Machado M, Tavares A, Ornellas AA, Molina WR, Juliano RV, Wroclawski ER. Video endoscopic inguinal lymphadenectomy: a new minimally invasive procedure for radical management of inguinal nodes in patients with penile squamous cell carcinoma. J Urol. 2007;177(3):953–8.
86. Hu J, Li H, Cui Y, Liu P, Zhou X, Liu L, et al. Comparison of clinical feasibility and oncological outcomes between video endoscopic and open inguinal lymphadenectomy for penile cancer. Medicine. 2019;98(22):e15862.

87. Elsamra SE, Poch MA. Robotic inguinal lymphadenectomy for penile cancer: the why, how, and what. Transl Androl Urol. 2017;6(5):826–32.
88. O'Brien JS, Perera M, Manning T, Bozin M, Cabarkapa S, Chen E, et al. Penile cancer: contemporary lymph node management. J Urol. 2017;197(6):1387–95.
89. Graafland NM, Moonen LMF, van Boven HH, van Werkhoven E, Kerst JM, Horenblas S. Inguinal recurrence following therapeutic lymphadenectomy for node positive penile carcinoma: outcome and implications for management. J Urol. 2011;185(3):888–94.
90. Winters BR, Kearns JT, Holt SK, Mossanen M, Lin DW, Wright JL. Is there a benefit to adjuvant radiation in stage III penile cancer after lymph node dissection? Findings from the National Cancer Database. Urol Oncol. 2018;36(3):92.e11–6.
91. Franks KN, Kancherla K, Sethugavalar B, Whelan P, Eardley I, Kiltie AE. Radiotherapy for node positive penile cancer: experience of the leeds teaching hospitals. J Urol. 2011;186(2):524–9.
92. Robinson R, Marconi L, MacPepple E, Hakenberg OW, Watkin N, Yuan Y, et al. Risks and benefits of adjuvant radiotherapy after inguinal lymphadenectomy in node-positive penile cancer: a systematic review by the European Association of Urology Penile Cancer Guidelines Panel. Eur Urol. 2018;74(1):76–83.
93. Lorenzo GD, Buonerba C, Federico P, Perdonà S, Aieta M, Rescigno P, et al. Cisplatin and 5-fluorouracil in inoperable, stage IV squamous cell carcinoma of the penis. BJU Int. 2012;110(11b):E661–6.
94. Eliason M, Bowen G, Bowen A, Hazard L, Samlowski W. Primary treatment of verrucous carcinoma of the penis with fluorouracil, cis-diamino-dichloro-platinum, and radiation therapy. Arch Dermatol. 2009;145(8):950–2.
95. Necchi A, Pond GR, Raggi D, Ottenhof SR, Djajadiningrat RS, Horenblas S, et al. Clinical outcomes of perioperative chemotherapy in patients with locally advanced penile squamous-cell carcinoma: results of a multicenter analysis. Clin Genitourin Canc. 2017;15(5):548–55.e3
96. Bandini M, Pederzoli F, Necchi A. Neoadjuvant chemotherapy for lymph node-positive penile cancer: current evidence and knowledge. Curr Opin Urol. 2020;30(2):218–22.
97. Lorenzo GD, Federico P, Buonerba C, Longo N, Cartenì G, Autorino R, et al. Paclitaxel in pretreated metastatic penile cancer: final results of a phase 2 study. Eur Urol. 2011;60(6):1280–4.
98. Power DG, Galvin DJ, Cuffe S, McVey GP, Mulholland PJ, Farrelly C, et al. Cisplatin and gemcitabine in the management of metastatic penile cancer. Urol Oncol. 2009;27(2):187–90.
99. Necchi A, Vullo SL, Mariani L, Zhu Y, Ye D-W, Ornellas AA, et al. Nomogram-based prediction of overall survival after regional lymph node dissection and the role of perioperative chemotherapy in penile squamous cell carcinoma: a retrospective multicenter study. Urol Oncol. 2019;37(8):531.e7–531.e15.
100. Noronha V, Patil V, Ostwal V, Tongaonkar H, Bakshi G, Prabhash K. Role of paclitaxel and platinum-based adjuvant chemotherapy in high-risk penile cancer. Urol Ann. 2012;4(3):150–3.

9 The Role of Chemotherapy and Radiotherapy in Penile Cancer

Constantine Alifrangis and Anita Mitra

Learning Objectives

After reading this chapter you will be able to:

- Discuss the indications of chemotherapy as a palliative treatment in metastatic penile cancer disease
- Explain the role of chemotherapy as neoadjuvant or adjuvant treatment in patients with locally advanced disease
- Describe potential uses of radiotherapy as a combination or primary treatment for patients with advanced or metastatic disease.
- Understand the importance of a multidisciplinary team in selecting appropriate combination therapies when managing penile cancer patients

Chemotherapy

Cytotoxic chemotherapy has been used as palliative treatment to prolong life and improve symptoms in metastatic inoperable penile cancer [1] and more recently has moved forward in the therapeutic algorithm as an important perioperative treatment in high risk locally advanced node positive disease. Traditionally deemed a malignancy with a chemo-resistant phenotype, penile squamous cell carcinoma has long been considered a challenging disease to treat for this reason.

C. Alifrangis (✉) · A. Mitra
Cancer Services, University College London Hospitals NHS Foundation Trust, London, UK
e-mail: constantine.alifrangis1@nhs.net

O. Brunckhorst et al. (eds.), *Penile Cancer – A Practical Guide*, Management of Urology, https://doi.org/10.1007/978-3-031-32681-3_9

Palliative Chemotherapy for Metastatic Disease

In the presence of metastatic disease palliative chemotherapy is offered to patients with a reasonable performance status (ECOG) of 2 or less. It is important to note that data to support these interventions is based on non-randomized data based on likely heterogeneous patient cohorts, usually from high volume institutional series.

Platinum based doublet chemotherapy is the backbone of therapy of metastatic disease with regimens often utilised that have been demonstrated to have activity in other genito-urinary or squamous cell malignancies. Older regimens such as Methotrexate and Bleomycin have been abandoned due toxicity concerns (Table 9.1) [1, 2]. The most commonly utilised approaches include cisplatin and infusional 5-Fluorouracil (5FU) [3] and platinum plus a taxane such as paclitaxel, being on the whole well tolerated outpatient regimens. The use of such regimens in penile squamous cell carcinoma (SCC) have been reported to have partial response or clinical benefit rates of between 20–40%, although profound responses have been reported. A UK Study of the triplet regimen Cisplatin 5fU and Docetaxel found a response rate of 38% with a common toxicity criteria (CTC) grade 3–4 toxicity rate of 63% [2]. A key phase II study demonstrating the ability to achieve a meaningful response with chemotherapy in this disease utilised Cisplatin, Paclitaxel and Ifosfamide (TIP) in a 3 day regimen every 21 days in the neoadjuvant treatment of inoperable disease and found a response rate of approximately 50% with a very acceptable toxicity profile [4]. Importantly about a 30% of patients were free of disease having undergone radical surgery at a median follow up of 34 months.

When selecting the most appropriate first line therapy for patients with metastatic disease most oncologists would consider the comorbidities and performance status of the patient. For example, if renal function is poor and there are vascular or

Table 9.1 Side effects of commonly utilised chemotherapy agents

Cisplatin	– Neutropenia and Thrombopenia – Nephrotoxicity and Neurotoxicity – Cardiotoxicity (Coronary spasms, ischaemia)
5-Fluorouracil	– Diarrhoea – Cardiotoxicity and Neurotoxicity
Paclitaxel	– Allergic Reactions – Alopecia
Ifosfamide	– Encephalopathy – Neurotoxicity and Nephrotoxicity – Haemorrhagic Cystitis – Diarrhoea
Methotrexate	– Pneumonitis and Fibrosis – Nephrotoxicity and Hepatoxicity – Toxic cutaneous reactions – Diarrhoea
Bleomycin	– Pneumonitis and Fibrosis – Raynaud Syndrome – Dermatitis

cardiac comorbidities cisplatin may not be appropriate, and carboplatin is often substituted in this setting as having a better cardiac and renal side effect profile. If the chemotherapy being given for distant metastatic disease e.g. thoracic metastases, i.e. with no prospect of downstaging to enable radical surgery, than doublet therapy is more likely to be appropriate with less toxicity than triplet regimens. Following failure of first line chemotherapy median survival in metastatic penile SCC is only 6–8 months. Clinical trial data in this setting is lacking. Single agent Paclitaxel given weekly as per gynaecological malignancies has been used in this setting as it is well tolerated [5], but no survival benefit has been demonstrated. A reasonable algorithm for metastatic disease for example as used in our institution may then include cisplatin or carboplatin plus 5FU first line and carboplatin paclitaxel or paclitaxel monotherapy as second line.

Neoadjuvant or Adjuvant Therapy for Locally Advanced Disease

In most other genitourinary malignancies, there is a clear mandate for intervention with systemic therapy in node positive locally advanced disease. In penile SCC the treatment of the regional lymph nodes has been controversial, and the benefit of chemotherapy in patients whose cancer has spread to regional lymph nodes less clear.

Studies have explored the efficacy of combination chemotherapy as neoadjuvant treatment before surgery for inoperable fixed or cN3 nodal disease [4, 6]. Initial data with triplet therapy revealed a response rate of up to 50% [4] and complete responses and surgical downstaging with some long-term responders also seen. EAU and NCCN guidance now reflects the clear mandate for intervention with a triplet regimen such as TIP or TPF in all eligible patients with locally advanced inoperable disease of the primary tumour or regional lymph nodes [7]. We would echo this recommendation and have seen dramatic responses in locally advanced disease, including in rarer disease subtypes such as posterior urethral SCC [8]. Most physicians have continued to advocate for the importance of this intervention through the COVID-19 pandemic and a recent consensus statement reflects this [9].

It is less clear what the right thing to do for patients who have had radical nodal clearance with high-risk disease (pN2-pN3)- ie multiple involved inguinal nodes or the presence of positive pelvic nodes or extranodal extension. The InPACT trial is a multicentre international collaboration hoping to establish in a randomised Bayesian trial design the standard of care for patients with locally advanced penile SCC, currently recruiting in Europe and the USA [10]. The data for utilising post-operative adjuvant chemotherapy has been based on small retrospective cohort studies [11, 12], however more recent multicentre studies did show improvements in progression free survival in the highest risk patients, including those with involved pelvic nodes [13]. Our network has recently published data showing that in those patients with highest risk disease features at surgery combination chemotherapy *and* radiotherapy offers improved disease-free survival (68%) compared to adjuvant radiotherapy alone (54%) compared to 29% for those patients who had no

Table 9.2 Summary of European Association of Urology Guidelines for chemotherapy in patients with penile cancer [7]

Recommendation	Strength rating
Patients with pN2-3 tumours should be offered adjuvant chemotherapy after radical lymphadenectomy. This should consist of three to four cycles of cisplatin, a taxane and 5-fluorouracil or ifosfamide.	Strong
In patients with non-resectable or recurrent lymph node metastases neoadjuvant chemotherapy should be offered. This should include four cycles of a cisplatin- and taxane-based regimen prior to radical surgery.	Weak
In palliative patients with systemic disease palliative chemotherapy should be offered.	Weak

adjuvant treatment (Alifrangis et al. presentation at ESMO 2020). However not all data is supportive. A recent study of data from a US National registry [14] suggested that receipt of adjuvant chemotherapy in node positive disease was not associated with improved overall survival on multivariate analysis. Although there continues to be a lack of prospective published data, adjuvant chemotherapy is recommended in EAU and NCCN guidance in high-risk node positive penile SCC (Table 9.2).

Immunotherapy

Given its status as a HPV driven tumour preclinical work has defined that Penile SCC expresses PDL1 and may be amenable to therapeutic intervention with PDl1 targeted immunotherapies that have been so successful in other genitourinary cancers [15].

Cemiplimab is a PDL1 therapeutic which has been FDA approved in cutaneous inoperable SCC following a landmark phase 2 trial with a response rate of 47% including in one patient with penile cancer. Although a malignancy with a different aetiology and pathogenesis, these cancers have a high tumour mutational burden (TMB) which can be prognostic of tumours that are more likely to respond to immunotherapy [16]. As a rare cancer, penile cancer trials are scarce hampering the evidence base for newer interventions, but some data is available from case series and phase II basket studies looking at rare cancers. Although there remains a paucity of data, responses with PDL1 immunotherapy such as pembrolizmab have been observed in metastatic penile cancer. Interestingly, in one cohort of two patients with high tumour mutational burden [17], and in another in a patient with Microsatellite instability or mismatch repair deficiency (MMR) [18]. Indeed, Pembrolizumab has achieved an FDA approval in a tumour agnostic setting given the responses seen across tumour types in patients with MMR repair deficiency [19]. The early data therefore suggests that although the response rate to immunotherapy is not high, it may be a useful strategy, even in chemo resistant disease in patients whose tumours have a genotype of TMB high or MMR Deficiency.

Radiotherapy

The role of radiation in the penile cancer has evolved, but because of its rarity, there is no level one evidence supporting its routine use. In clinical practice however, it is used in the neoadjuvant, adjuvant and primary settings and in both radical and palliative treatment.

The management of penile cancer is divided into the treatment of the primary lesion within the penis and then consideration of the lymphatic drainage. As discussed in Chap. 8 the nodal spread is stepwise in progression and nodal staging forms an important part of subsequent management. The lymph node status has a significant effect on overall survival with the likelihood of pelvic lymph node disease increasing with the number of positive inguinal lymph nodes. The potential risk of pelvic nodal disease is 16–23% with 2 positive inguinal nodes and 44–56% with extracapsular spread or more than 3 lymph nodes [20, 21]. The 5-year survival in lymph node negative disease is 95%, 76% when only inguinal lymph nodes are positive and as low as zero when pelvic nodes are involved in some studies [22].

Most of the radiation used in the management of penile cancer is delivered using external beam radiation, brachytherapy is used less commonly.

External Beam Radiotherapy Using Intensity Modulated Radiation

Radiotherapy uses high energy radiation beams using x-rays, also called photons, and are delivered from a machine called a linear accelerator. It works by damaging tumour cells in the treated body part. The radiation stops the cells from dividing and growing. Radiotherapy can also damage nearby normal cells. The normal cells are more likely to recover from the effects of the radiation than the cancer or tumour cells. The photon beams are shaped using lead leaflets to reduce the amount of radiation that is received by the normal tissues.

It is administered as an outpatient procedure for around 60–90 min per day and in the radical (curative) setting may be over 5 weeks, Monday to Friday (25 fractions or 25 days of treatment). The patient needs to be able to lie still independently on the treatment couch and be compliant with bladder and bowel preparation instructions. The treatment is planned on a CT scan and then this is used to project the beams of radiation and create a dose distribution. This can be administered with concomitant chemotherapy.

Radiotherapy delivery is very similar to having an x-ray taken and patients are not radioactive after treatment, and are safe to be around family, friends, and pregnant women. The side effects generally start 2 weeks into the treatment and include tiredness, skin changes and pain and swelling and changes in bowel habit. The addition of chemotherapy can make the side effects worse and may cause nausea and vomiting. Long term, there may be skin changes, loss of pubic hair, long term bowel changes and lymphoedema of the legs or scrotum.

Table 9.3 Common side effects of penile brachytherapy

Short Term	– Dermatitis, hypopigmentation and telangiectasia – Sterile Urethritis – Adhesions in the Urethra
Long Term	– Soft Tissue Necrosis—Particularly T3 tumours and higher volume implants – Delayed healing/tissue ulceration – Meatal Stenosis

Brachytherapy

Brachytherapy is the insertion of radioactive needles, or sources directly in or near the tumour. It requires circumcision to take place before the procedure in some instances. The implants give off radiation over a short period of time and over a short distance. The needles are lined up so that they cover the tumour and a margin around it. The radiation is administered once or twice daily over several days. Once the sources are removed from the body after each treatment, the patient is not radioactive.

Radiation side effects (Table 9.3) are broken down into short term (during the treatment, usually reversible taking 2–3 months to heal) and long term (after the treatment; this may be months or years afterwards). Erectile function is usually maintained because the erectile tissues including the penile shaft and corpora do not receive a significant amount of radiation [23].

Adjuvant Radiotherapy to the Pelvis

The use of adjuvant radiation is a debated area. The aim of this treatment with or without concomitant cisplatin is to improve the local control rate of the disease and therefore quality of life, to also impact on overall survival potentially. The rationale for the treatment comes from the observation of local disease recurrence in those men with positive inguinal lymph nodes treated with lymphadenectomy alone. Recurrence rates have been reported as being between 25–75% [24, 25].

There is concern regarding radiation toxicity and the benefit of treatment. As a result, recent EAU guidelines do not recommend the routine use of adjuvant radiation outside of a clinical trial. A recent systematic review [26] of reported adjuvant radiotherapy studies in node positive penile cancer found no good evidence of a survival benefit. The literature is small, often retrospective and mixes patients who were treated radically and palliatively together. The data often do not record the dose of radiation received and administration methods. Up to date radiation techniques such as Intensity Modulated Radiation are rarely used.

Ager et al. publishing in 2021 have reviewed a single institution outcome of 121 patients who were treated with adjuvant radiotherapy in the post-operative setting for pN3 disease. Of the 55 patients that recurred 30 were in the pelvic and inguinal area, 26 of whom were within the radiation field. 18 patients relapsed in visceral sites. This suggests a local control rate in the region of 75% in this cohort. The 5-year RFS was 51%, CSS was 51% and OS was 44% [27]. The radiation dose and administration were using up to date radiotherapy techniques. The outcomes for this group of patients are better than recorded historically for pN3 disease, which has meant that similar centres persist in the use of adjuvant radiation in higher risk disease despite EAU guidance [7]. Prior to this publication, two series reported on the use of adjuvant radiation in those men with greater than or equal to 2 lymph nodes positive in the groin or the presence of extracapsular spread [24, 28]. In both studies, the outcomes were better than predicted from case series that did not have adjuvant radiation.

Neoadjuvant Radiotherapy to the Pelvis

The use of radiation often along with cisplatin (concomitant chemoradiation) is in routine use where inguinal disease is inoperable or where the patient is not fit enough for radical surgery. The aim of this is to downstage the disease to make it operable or to deliver radical (curative) radiation. There are no data to support its use, but the intention is to attempt to control the disease locoregionally and so improve quality of life and potentially to improve overall survival and to improve operability. This is borne of the difficulty in managing untreated local disease that fungates, causing pain, bleeding, and sepsis. The role of neoadjuvant chemoradiotherapy is being examined in the previously mentioned InPACT study [10].

Primary Radiotherapy to the Penis

Advances in penile preserving and surgical reconstructive techniques have meant that radiation to the primary lesion is unusual. Surgery also enables pelvic lymph node management [29].

External beam radiotherapy can provide an alternative to surgery with a reasonable chance of control of the disease. There have been only a few series that have reported the outcomes of men treated with external beam radiation and local failure is more likely with higher grade disease, lesions that are greater than T3, disease that receives less than 60Gy and less than 2Gy per fraction treated over more than 45 days [29].

Brachytherapy has been reported to show good control rates in selected cases. Lesions that are of clinical stage T1b or T2 and less than 4 cm in maximum diameter may be considered for primary brachytherapy. Lesions confined to the glans are ideal but those with minor extension across the coronal sulcus may also be treated provided the extension can be covered with an additional plane of needles. Tumours that extend into the penile urethra are not suitable for brachytherapy, because of the dose delivered to the urethra [23].

Palliative Radiation

Where penile cancer is too advanced to be operable or the fitness of the individual precludes surgery, palliative radiation may be considered. There is no standard method if radiation or chemoradiation is used to downstage disease to make it operable (see above). If disease recurs or if loco-regional disease in the pelvis is causing symptoms in the situation where it has also metastasised outside of the body, palliative radiation may be an option to regain some local control. Palliative radiation is also used to treat painful bone metastases and chest lesions which may be causing breathing difficulties or venous occlusion. The courses of treatment are generally short and have few side effects.

Conclusion

Chemotherapy and radiation may in summary be used in many instances in the management of this rare malignancy, in some cases there is emerging data that these can be lifesaving interventions in a disease with an aggressive natural history. We would advocate that best practice is to involve oncologists early in the pathway of the patient and ensure multidisciplinary decision making.

Key Points

- Chemotherapy forms the backbone of the management of palliative management in metastatic penile cancer
- Chemotherapy has an important role in the neoadjuvant or adjuvant setting in those with high risk, locally advanced disease
- External Beam Radiotherapy using Intensity Modulated Radiation and brachytherapy can play an important role as a combination therapy in palliative patients or those with high-risk disease
- Appropriate expertise within the penile cancer multidisciplinary team is important to enable the selection of appropriate combination therapies for individual patients

Test your learning and check your understanding of this book's contents: use the "Springer Nature Flashcards" app to access questions using ▶ https://sn.pub/1r7Om8. To use the app, please follow the instructions in chapter 1.

References

1. Protzel C, Hakenberg OW. Chemotherapy in patients with penile carcinoma. Urol Int. 2009;82(1):1–7.
2. Nicholson S, Hall E, Harland SJ, Chester JD, Pickering L, Barber J, et al. Phase II trial of docetaxel, cisplatin and 5FU chemotherapy in locally advanced and metastatic penis cancer (CRUK/09/001). Br J Cancer. 2013;109(10):2554–9.

3. Shammas FV, Ous S, Fossa SD. Cisplatin and 5-fluorouracil in advanced cancer of the penis. J Urol. 1992;147(3):630–2.
4. Pagliaro LC, Williams DL, Daliani D, Williams MB, Osai W, Kincaid M, et al. Neoadjuvant paclitaxel, ifosfamide, and cisplatin chemotherapy for metastatic penile cancer: a phase II study. J Clin Oncol. 2010;28(24):3851–7.
5. Di Lorenzo G, Carteni G, Autorino R, Gonnella A, Perdona S, Ferro M, et al. Activity and toxicity of paclitaxel in pretreated metastatic penile cancer patients. Anti-Cancer Drugs. 2009;20(4):277–80.
6. Bermejo C, Busby JE, Spiess PE, Heller L, Pagliaro LC, Pettaway CA. Neoadjuvant chemotherapy followed by aggressive surgical consolidation for metastatic penile squamous cell carcinoma. J Urol. 2007;177(4):1335–8.
7. Hakenberg OW, Comperat EM, Minhas S, Necchi A, Protzel C, Watkin N. EAU guidelines on penile cancer: 2014 update. Eur Urol. 2015;67(1):142–50.
8. Castiglione F, Alnajjar HM, Christodoulidou M, Albersen M, Parnham A, Freeman A, et al. Primary squamous cell carcinoma of the male proximal urethra: outcomes from a single centre. Eur Urol Focus. 2021;7(1):163–9.
9. Cakir OO, Castiglione F, Tandogdu Z, Collins J, Alnajjar HM, Akers C, et al. Management of penile cancer patients during the COVID-19 pandemic: an eUROGEN accelerated Delphi consensus study. Urol Oncol. 2021;39(3):197. e9- e17
10. Canter DJ, Nicholson S, Watkin N, Hall E, Pettaway C, In PEC. The international penile advanced cancer trial (InPACT): rationale and current status. Eur Urol Focus. 2019;5(5):706–9.
11. Pizzocaro G, Piva L, Bandieramonte G, Tana S. Up-to-date management of carcinoma of the penis. Eur Urol. 1997;32(1):5–15.
12. Hakenberg OW, Nippgen JB, Froehner M, Zastrow S, Wirth MP. Cisplatin, methotrexate and bleomycin for treating advanced penile carcinoma. BJU Int. 2006;98(6):1225–7.
13. Sharma P, Djajadiningrat R, Zargar-Shoshtari K, Catanzaro M, Zhu Y, Nicolai N, et al. Adjuvant chemotherapy is associated with improved overall survival in pelvic node-positive penile cancer after lymph node dissection: a multi-institutional study. Urol Oncol. 2015;33(11):496. e17-23
14. Joshi SS, Handorf E, Strauss D, Correa AF, Kutikov A, Chen DYT, et al. Treatment trends and outcomes for patients with lymph node-positive cancer of the penis. JAMA Oncol. 2018;4(5):643–9.
15. Cocks M, Taheri D, Ball MW, Bezerra SM, Del Carmen Rodriguez M, Ricardo BFP, et al. Immune-checkpoint status in penile squamous cell carcinoma: a North American cohort. Hum Pathol. 2017;59:55–61.
16. Migden MR, Rischin D, Schmults CD, Guminski A, Hauschild A, Lewis KD, et al. PD-1 blockade with Cemiplimab in advanced cutaneous squamous-cell carcinoma. N Engl J Med. 2018;379(4):341–51.
17. Chahoud J, Skelton WPT, Spiess PE, Walko C, Dhillon J, Gage KL, et al. Case report: two cases of chemotherapy refractory metastatic penile squamous cell carcinoma with extreme durable response to pembrolizumab. Front Oncol. 2020;10:615298.
18. Hahn AW, Chahoud J, Campbell MT, Karp DD, Wang J, Stephen B, et al. Pembrolizumab for advanced penile cancer: a case series from a phase II basket trial. Investig New Drugs. 2021;39(5):1405–10.
19. Marcus L, Lemery SJ, Keegan P, Pazdur R. FDA approval summary: pembrolizumab for the treatment of microsatellite instability-high solid tumors. Clin Cancer Res. 2019;25(13):3753–8.
20. Lont AP, Kroon BK, Gallee MP, van Tinteren H, Moonen LM, Horenblas S. Pelvic lymph node dissection for penile carcinoma: extent of inguinal lymph node involvement as an indicator for pelvic lymph node involvement and survival. J Urol. 2007;177(3):947–52. discussion 52
21. Ornellas AA, Seixas AL, Marota A, Wisnescky A, Campos F, de Moraes JR. Surgical treatment of invasive squamous cell carcinoma of the penis: retrospective analysis of 350 cases. J Urol. 1994;151(5):1244–9.
22. Ravi R. Morbidity following groin dissection for penile carcinoma. Br J Urol. 1993;72(6):941–5.
23. Crook JM, Haie-Meder C, Demanes DJ, Mazeron JJ, Martinez AA, Rivard MJ. American Brachytherapy Society-Groupe Europeen de Curietherapie-European Society of Therapeutic Radiation Oncology (ABS-GEC-ESTRO) consensus statement for penile brachytherapy. Brachytherapy. 2013;12(3):191–8.

24. Culkin DJ, Beer TM. Advanced penile carcinoma. J Urol. 2003;170(2 Pt 1):359–65.
25. Ozsahin M, Jichlinski P, Weber DC, Azria D, Zimmermann M, Guillou L, et al. Treatment of penile carcinoma: to cut or not to cut? Int J Radiat Oncol Biol Phys. 2006;66(3):674–9.
26. Robinson R, Marconi L, MacPepple E, Hakenberg OW, Watkin N, Yuan Y, et al. Risks and benefits of adjuvant radiotherapy after inguinal lymphadenectomy in node-positive penile cancer: a systematic review by the European Association of Urology penile cancer guidelines panel. Eur Urol. 2018;74(1):76–83.
27. Ager M, Njoku K, Serra M, Robinson A, Pickering L, Afshar M, et al. Long-term multicentre experience of adjuvant radiotherapy for pN3 squamous cell carcinoma of the penis. BJU Int. 2021;128(4):451–9.
28. Franks KN, Kancherla K, Sethugavalar B, Whelan P, Eardley I, Kiltie AE. Radiotherapy for node positive penile cancer: experience of the Leeds teaching hospitals. J Urol. 2011;186(2):524–9.
29. Van Poppel H, Watkin NA, Osanto S, Moonen L, Horwich A, Kataja V, et al. Penile cancer: ESMO clinical practice guidelines for diagnosis, treatment and follow-up. Ann Oncol. 2013;24(Suppl 6):vi115-24.

Reconstructive Surgical Techniques in Penile Cancer

10

Laura Elst, Wai Gin Lee, and Maarten Albersen

Learning Objectives
After reading this chapter you will be able to:

- Identify indications and options for organ sparing and reconstructive treatments in patients with penile cancer
- Recognise the functional and aesthetic advantages of organ sparing approaches
- Explain the surgical technique for utilised organ sparing and reconstructive options, including grafting techniques
- Understand the importance of careful patient selection and strict surveillance protocols when considering these techniques

Introduction

The surgical treatment of penile cancer is strongly dependent on the pathological stage and location of the tumour [1]. The pathological stage is currently defined by the American Joint Committee on Cancer (AJCC) and the Union Internationale Contre le Cancer (UICC) TNM clinical classification system (eighth edition) as discussed in more detail in Chap. 4. These facilitate the prediction of prognosis and therefore the choice of definitive treatment [2].

L. Elst · M. Albersen (✉)
Department of Urology, University Hospitals Leuven, Leuven, Belgium
e-mail: maarten.albersen@uzleuven.be

W. G. Lee
Department of Urology, University College London Hospitals NHS Foundation Trust, London, UK

O. Brunckhorst et al. (eds.), *Penile Cancer – A Practical Guide*, Management of Urology, https://doi.org/10.1007/978-3-031-32681-3_10

Surgery has always played a central role in the treatment of penile cancer, both for eradication of the primary tumour and for obtaining definitive diagnosis and staging. Previously surgical excision of the primary tumour with a 2 cm margin was the gold standard [3, 4]. However, consequences following radical penectomy, which include the inability to pass urine in an upright position and loss of sexual function, are debilitating for patients [5]. Moreover, a significant reduction of penile length and the loss of penile function, appearance and sensation cause significant morbidity and a reduction in quality of life if partial penectomy is chosen. Therefore, there has been a shift to less-invasive surgical strategies to improve quality of life and penile function. When oncologically feasible, organ-sparing surgery (OSS) is preferred [6]. In principle, all tumours that are not invading into the corpus cavernosum are potential candidates for OSS and even if only the tip, or tunica involvement is present, reconstructive options are available [7]. A disadvantage of using OSS, is the higher risk of local recurrence, although several studies have proven that local recurrence has little influence on long-term survival [8, 9]. Moreover, clear resection margins of less than 5 mm, and even as low as 1 mm, seem to be safe and do not influence oncological outcome [9, 10]. However, there remains debate in the subject with a recent study challenging the use of OSS by demonstrating that local recurrence after upfront glansectomy was strongly associated with worse overall survival (OS) and cancer specific survival (CSS) in higher grade tumours [11]. Hence, the recommendation for the use of OSS differs between guidelines with the NCCN advocating it's use only in lower grade and stage lesions whereas the EAU recommends to perform OSS "whenever possible" [12, 13]. OSS is currently a widely accepted treatment method for distal penile cancer. In addition, many patients are eligible, provided that approximately 80% of patients develop penile cancer on the prepuce and/or glans [11].

In this chapter we aim to describe reconstructive surgical techniques, which can be used after surgical resection of primary penile tumours. Surgical treatment options used in inguinal or pelvic nodal metastatic disease are beyond the scope of this chapter and are instead covered in Chap. 7 of this book.

Indications

Surgical options for penile sparing treatments include circumcision, wide local excision, glans resurfacing, partial glansectomy and glansectomy. The extent of tumour invasion in the corpora will determine between the use of OSS, partial penectomy and total penectomy [4]. Regarding predictive pathological risk factors, careful selection of patients is crucial when making treatment decisions. Even more important is patient counselling and a good understanding of patient's expectations in comparison with realistic treatment options. In addition, patients must be compliant to follow-up when considering OSS. Common indications for different OSS options are discussed in more detail in Table 10.1.

Table 10.1 Indications and Surgical Options for Penile Sparing Treatments by Stage of Disease. European Association of Urology (EAU) guidelines on penile cancer [5, 12], National Comprehensive Cancer Network (NCCN) guidelines on penile cancer [13]

Penile cancer stage – grade	Surgical treatment options (EAU guidelines)	Surgical treatment options (NCCN guidelines)
PeIN	Wide local excision/ circumcision Glans resurfacing Glansectomy, partial glansectomy	Wide local excision/ circumcision Glans resurfacing Total glansectomy
pTa pT1a (G1, G2)	Wide local excision/ circumcision Glans resurfacing Glansectomy, partial glansectomy	Wide local excision/ circumcision Total glansectomy Partial penectomy
pT1b (G3)	Wide local excision/ circumcision Glansectomy, partial glansectomy	Wide local excision/ circumcision Total glansectomy Partial penectomy Total penectomy
pT2	Wide local excision with circumcision Glansectomy Partial penectomy	Partial penectomy Total penectomy
T3 (treatment of disease invading the corpora cavernosa and/or urethra.)	Glansectomy with distal corporectomy Partial penectomy Total penectomy with reconstruction of the urethra	Partial penectomy Total penectomy with reconstruction of the urethra
pT4 (Treatment of locally advanced disease invading adjacent structures.)	Partial penectomy Total penectomy with perineal urethrostomy	Partial penectomy Total penectomy with perineal urethrostomy

Surgical Techniques

Wide Local Excision and Circumcision

Wide local excision or circumcision can be offered for local disease, depending on the location and extent of the tumour. PeIN and pT1 tumours confined to the prepuce can be treated by circumcision in which resection of preputial skin, as widely as necessary to achieve negative margins, is performed [14]. Although radical circumcision may potentially result in sensation changes of the glans, it is an essential element in the surgical treatment of penile cancer [15].

If the lesion invades the glans (usually the corona) as well, radical circumcision with wide local excision can be conducted. Skin lesions can be closed primarily or reconstruction is performed according to the tissue defect [14]. For lesions on the corona, a preputial advancement flap can prove helpful.

For patients with distal urethral lesions, surgical excision is required, followed by reconstruction of a neomeatus or neourethra. In cases of extensive excision of the distal urethra, urethroplasty with skin grafts or buccal mucosa, can be performed [3, 5].

Glans Resurfacing and Split-Thickness Skin Graft (STSG)

Glans resurfacing is a surgical technique indicated for local disease: peIN and pT1a. Historically it was developed by Bracka for the surgical treatment of considerable cases of lichen sclerosus et atrophicans (LS) [5]. Nowadays glans resurfacing is also used for localized and superficial tumours of the glans. This technique realizes excision of the epithelium and subepithelium, which is a less extensive surgical technique compared to glansectomy [14]. If less than 50% of the glans is involved, partial glans resurfacing is an appropriate alternative. As such, the preservation of the corona for sensation has recently been described [16]. Glans resurfacing can be offered as a treatment method for patients with in-situ malignancy, who failed topical treatment or who are unwilling to follow strict surveillance protocols, as recurrence rates are low since the complete glans epithelium is extirpated [5, 17, 18].

Surgical Technique

This technique is performed preferably under a general anaesthetic as multiple operative fields are involved, and handling of grafts can be delicate so patient movement is to be avoided [17]. Broad spectrum antibiotics are administered preoperatively [19]. First, in uncircumcised patients, a circumcision is performed, and the penis is partially degloved. After applying a tourniquet at the shaft or base of the penis, the glans skin is marked in four quadrants from the meatus to the coronal sulcus. Afterwards, the tip of each quadrant is lifted, starting at the meatus. The plane is easier to identify in cases where no previous treatments were performed and in cases with PeIN only with no invasive components. The glans epithelium and subepithelium are dissected from the meatus to the coronal sulcus (Fig. 10.1). After the dissection of glans tissue is completed, it is advised to remove the tourniquet, which allows to identify and control excessive bleeding which can be coagulated using bipolar energy. Venous oozing usually stops when the graft is applied.

A split-thickness skin graft is then harvested preferably from the thigh, at the level where the donor site is not visible in swimming trunks, within a dermatome and is used to cover the glans (Fig. 10.2) [17]. A graft thickness of 0.016 to 0.018 inches is robust to work with, does not compromise graft take and is the standard in our centre. In case of smoking, vascular disease or diabetes, graft healing can be compromised, therefore the use of grafts should be discouraged in severe vascular disease, uncontrolled diabetes or when the patient refuses to quit smoking. Absorbable quilting sutures with monofilament poliglecaprone 5.0 are used (Fig. 10.3). Small cuts can be made through the graft to evacuate

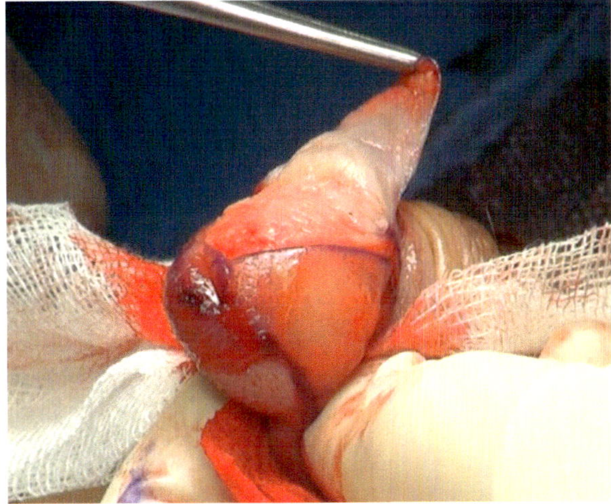

Fig. 10.1 The glans epithelium and subepithelium of each quadrant are dissected from the meatus to the coronal sulcus to remove the tumour

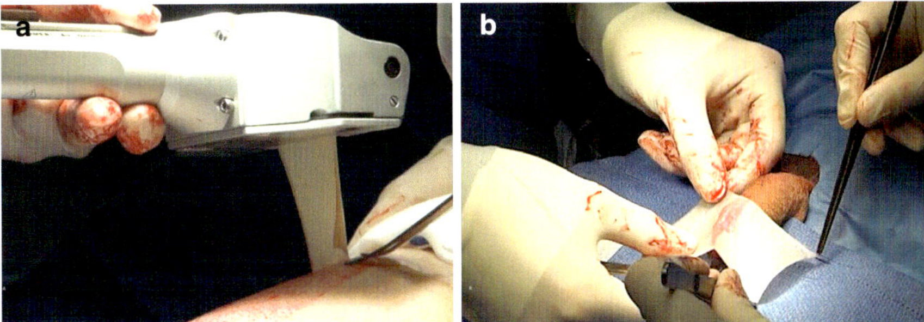

Fig. 10.2 (**a**, **b**) An air-powered dermatome is used to harvest the STSG from the thigh. The STSG is used to cover the spongious tissue of the glans

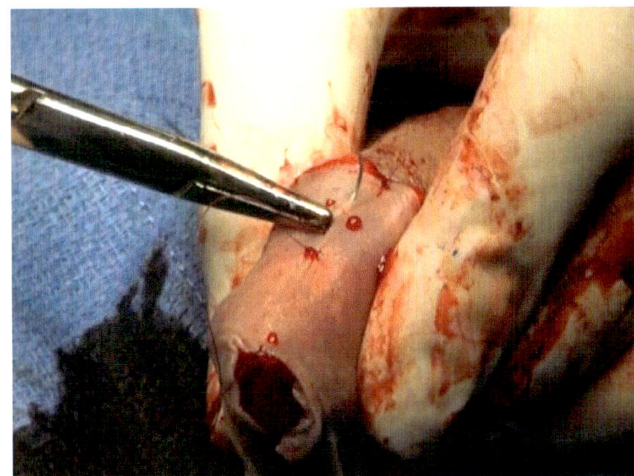

Fig. 10.3 The extragenital STSG is applied over the corpora and the neoglans is quilted with monofilament 5.0 sutures, which compresses the graft to its bed and reduces potential space for hematoma formation

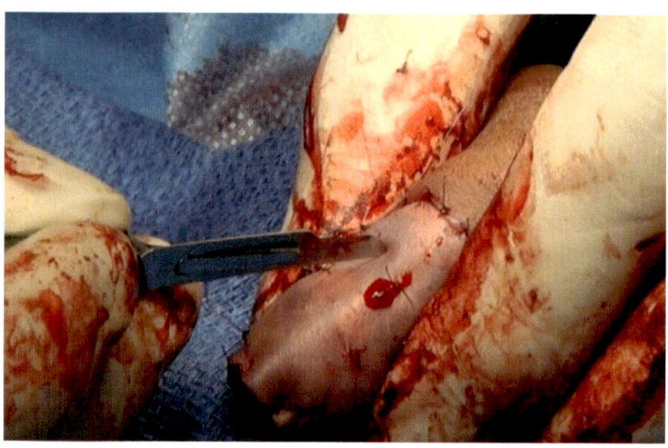

Fig. 10.4 Small cuts in the graft are made with the tip of a no. 15 blade in order to evacuate the hematoma under the graft

any hematoma under the graft using a blade or hypodermic needle (Fig. 10.4). Meshing can also be employed but can pose challenges in control of bleeding. The patient is then catheterized and a paraffin soaked dressing is applied and sutured in place [20]. The catheter and dressing are left in place for 5–10 days. A penile anaesthetic block can be used for pain control for a few hours after surgery.

In general, this procedure allows for acceptable aesthetic outcomes and penile function is largely preserved although a substantial proportion of patients report diminished sensation [19]. There is a relatively small risk of complications such as compromised graft take and infection compared to glansectomy, due to the well perfused graft bed [5]. Glans resurfacing provides complete histopathological analysis of the whole skin of the glans, which enables adequate staging of superficial penile cancer and PeIN. Up to 20% of patients with extensive PeIN are upstaged to invasive or micro-invasive disease on final pathology. Local recurrence is reported to occur in between 0% and 6% of patients [3, 21].

Split-Thickness Skin Graft (STSG) Harvesting, Application, and Wound Care

A STSG includes the epidermis and a variable amount of dermis. The donor site is selected depending on the characteristics of the surgical defect, including colour, texture, and thickness. Most often, the thigh is selected for STSG of genital lesions. Firstly, when harvesting STSG, the thigh is cleaned and prepared using liquid paraffin for lubrification [22]. Afterwards the STSG is harvested from the thigh with an air-powered dermatome [17] (Fig. 10.2a). Graft thickness ranges from 0.008 to 0.018 inches. In case of smoking, vascular disease or diabetes, graft healing can be compromised. Therefore, the use of grafts should be discouraged in severe vascular disease, uncontrolled diabetes or when the patient refuses to quit smoking. After the graft is sutured (Fig. 10.5), a tie-over dressing is applied to provide gentle pressure and compress the graft against the graft bed (Fig. 10.6a) [20, 22]. An

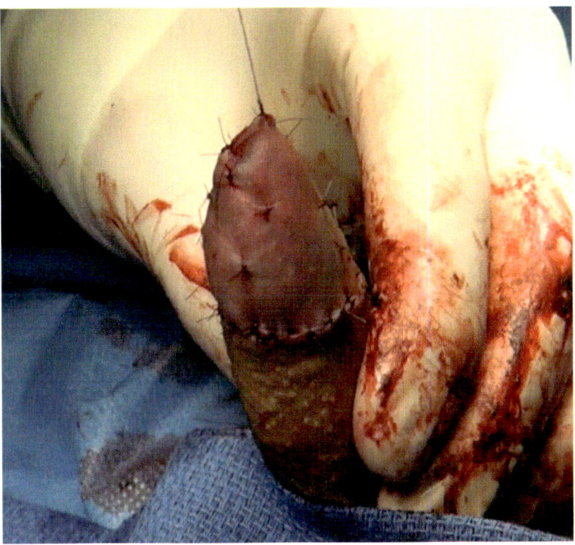

Fig. 10.5 Appearance of a STSG after application and quilting

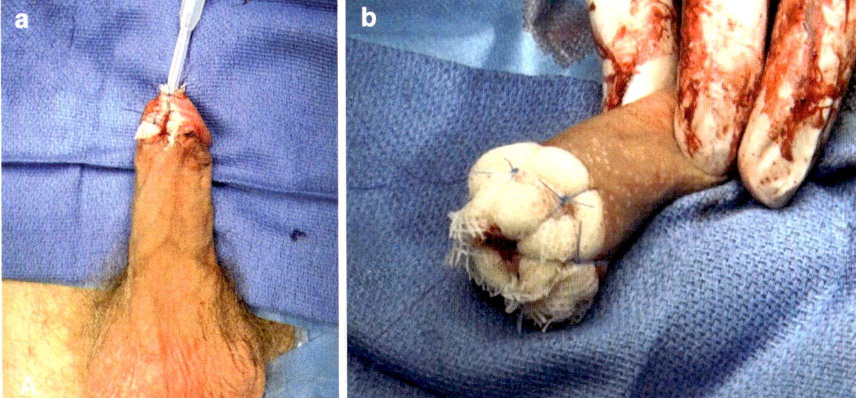

Fig. 10.6 (**a**) Tie-over dressing to compress the graft against the graft bed (**b**) Tie-over dressing consisting of silicone gauze and multiple layers of paraffin gauze

adherent dressing consisting of silicone gauze and multiple layers of paraffin gauze is applied to reduce sheer, which allows the patient to mobilize immediately after surgery (Fig. 10.6b) [22, 23]. After application of the dressing, a catheter is inserted.

The donor site on the thigh is infiltrated with 1% lidocaine and 1:200,000 adrenaline, which optimizes haemostasis and then covered with a calcium alginate dressing [22]. As there remains dermis, the donor site will heal spontaneously and in many cases, no obvious scar will be visible in the long term (Fig. 10.7) [23]. However, an area of altered pigmentation can occur.

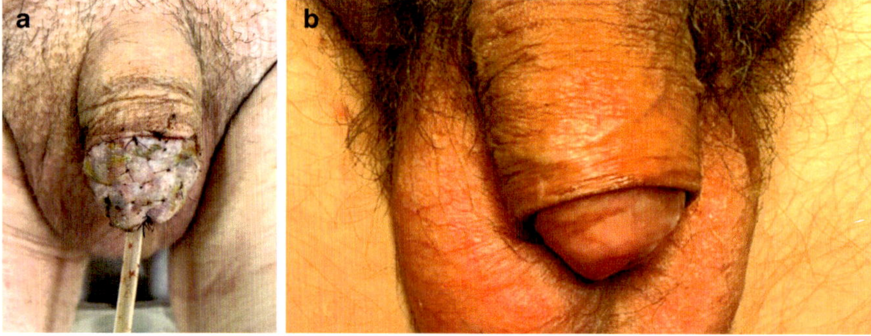

Fig. 10.7 (**a**) Appearance of STSG after removal of the tie-over dressing one-week post-operative. (**b**) Appearance of STSG 3 months post-operative

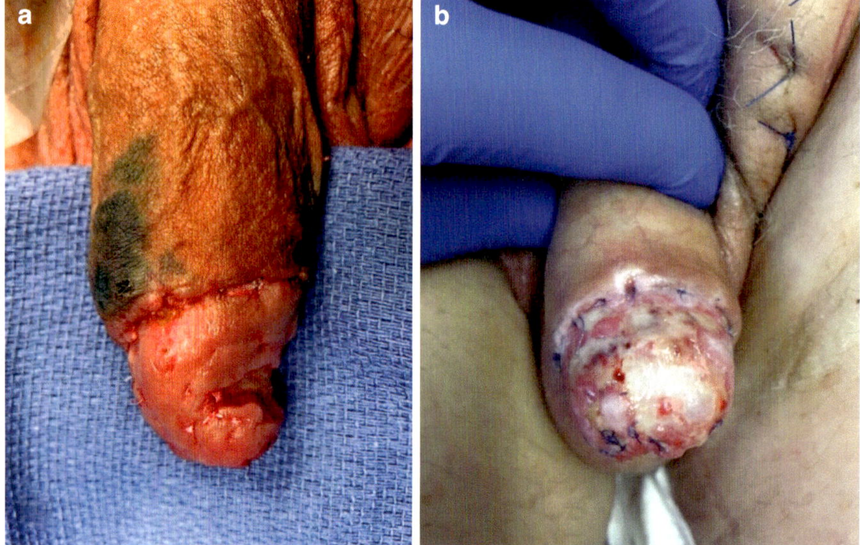

Fig. 10.8 (**a**) Example of partial failure of STSG. This lesion will heal spontaneously by granulation of tissue. (**b**) Example of subtotal failure of STSG, due to the avascular graft bed or infection after a glansectomy

The catheter and dressing are left in place for 5–10 days. Broad spectrum antibiotics are continued until the dressing is removed, as it is assumed that infection is one of the major causes of graft failure (Fig. 10.8a, b) [22].

Glansectomy

A glansectomy is indicated for locally advanced disease, located distally at the glans penis. Austoni et al. affirmed that the corpora cavernosa of the penis represent a well-defined anatomical structure distinct from the corpus spongiosum and the glans [24]. Removal of the glans spongiosum from the cavernosal heads is a surgical treatment option for T2 tumours and high grade T1 tumours [5]. Careful examination of the penile lesion is required to certify that the lesion is confined to the glans only. In case of doubt and when there is suspicion of more extensive invasion in the corpora cavernosa, preoperative imaging is required. In this case magnetic resonance imaging (MRI) of the penis in an erect state is performed [22]. Depending on the extent of tumour invasion, glansectomy is performed over versus under Buck's fascia. For cases with suspicion of corporal tip involvement, dissection under Buck's fascia is preferable and a distal corporectomy can be considered [14]. In smaller tumours, involving less than 50% of the glans: partial glansectomy and wide local excision are appropriate. In this cases the glans can be primarily closed or larger lesions can be covered by split-thickness skin grafts, full-thickness penile skin grafts or buccal mucosa grafts (BMG) [14].

Surgical Technique

This technique is usually performed under general anaesthetic and penile block. Broad spectrum antibiotics are administered preoperatively.

Surgical Technique Using Dissection over Buck's Fascia

In cases where tumour invasion is confined to the glans and not invading the corporal tips, dissection over Buck's fascia is advised. This protects the components of the dorsal neurovascular bundle. Additionally, a well vascularized bed, which optimizes graft taking is preserved. A potential detriment is having limited oncological safety margins.

First, a subcoronal skin incision is made (Fig. 10.9). Afterwards the plane between the glans and Buck's fascia is dissected. The dissection continues until the entire glans is dissected of the corporal heads and only the urethra remains intact. Bipolar diathermy is required for a meticulous haemostasis of this well vascularized anatomical region due to the small side arteries of the dorsal artery to the glans (Fig. 10.10). Finally, the urethra is transected below the tumour and

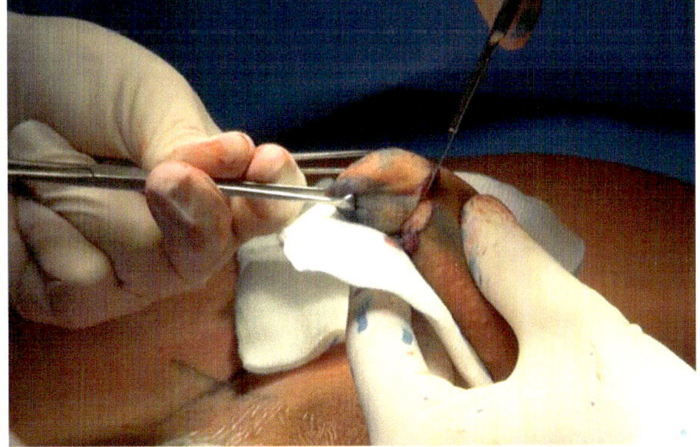

Fig. 10.9 Subcoronal skin incision. In uncircumcised men a circumcision is performed

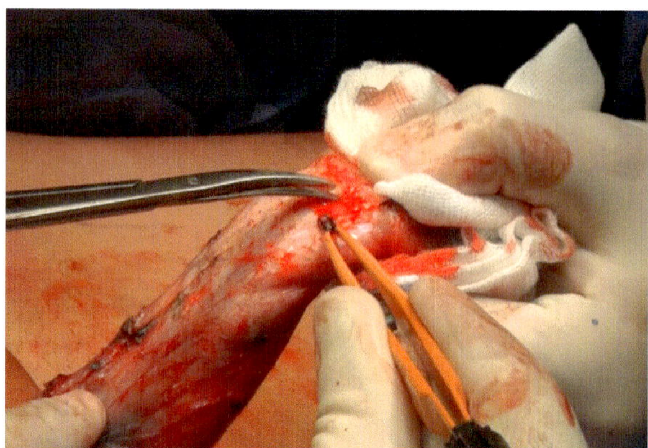

Fig. 10.10 Dissection over Buck's fascia. A thorough haemostasis is achieved by bipolar diathermy

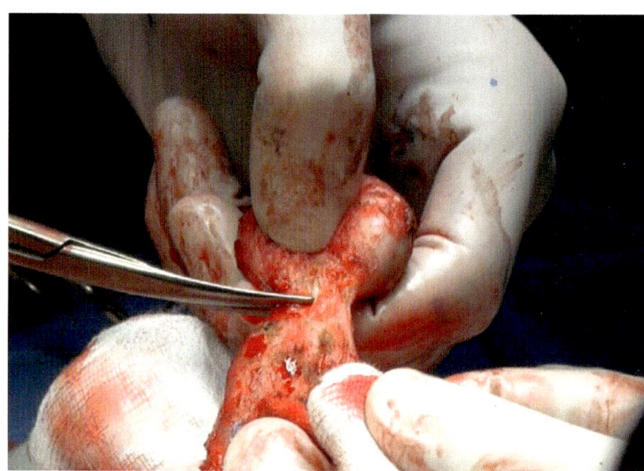

Fig. 10.11 The dissection continues until the entire glans is dissected of the corporal heads and only the urethra remains intact. Finally, the urethra is transected and placed within the corpora cavernosa

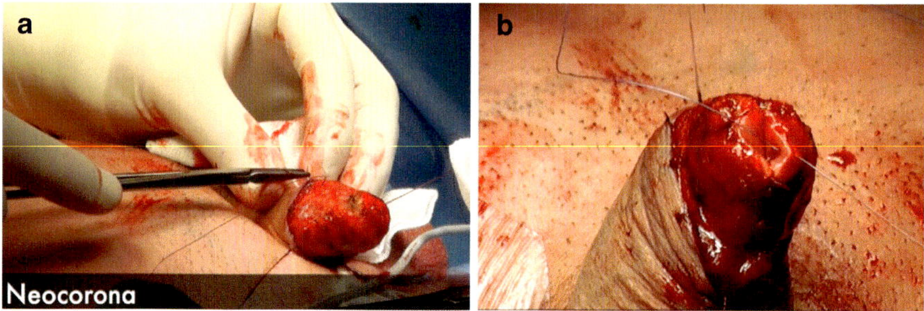

Fig. 10.12 (**a, b**) The urethra is spatulated and fixed to the corpora. Afterwards the penile shaft skin is sutured to the tunica albuginea of the underlying corporal bodies with 4.0 polyglactin sutures, forming a neoglans

splayed onto the cavernosal tips (Fig. 10.11). Suturing of the urethra to the corpora is sufficient in case of a good lumen (Fig. 10.12a) [22]. The penile shaft skin is sutured to the tunica albuginea of the underlying corporal bodies with 4.0 polyglactin sutures [7, 22]. Thereby a 2.5–3 cm gap is preserved, creating a neoglans (Fig. 10.12b).

Afterwards a STSG is harvested from the thigh to cover the neoglans, analogous to glans resurfacing technique. The STSG is fixed to the underlying Buck's fascia with quilting 5.0 monofilament sutures. The urethra is sutured to the graft with polyglactin 5.0 sutures, thereby avoid full-thickness sutures through the urethra to prevent fistula formation [22].

Post-operative dressing and management are identical to glans resurfacing. Broad spectrum antibiotics are continued for 7 days, as infection of the wound bed is an important cause of graft failure and neovascularization takes 5–7 days [22].

Surgical Technique Using Dissection under Buck's Fascia

In case of high-risk tumours and suspicion of corporal tip involvement, dissection under Buck's fascia, resulting in wider oncological margins, is advised. As the tunica albuginea is avascular, this technique contains the risk of having worse graft takes compared to classic dissection.

First, a subcoronal skin incision is made. The plane between the glans and Buck's fascia is dissected longitudinally. After Buck's fascia is dissected circumferentially, the neurovascular bundle is dissected from the tunica albuginea and ligated (Fig. 10.13). The dissection continues until Buck's fascia is dissected of the corporal heads and only the urethra remains attached. Further surgical technique is

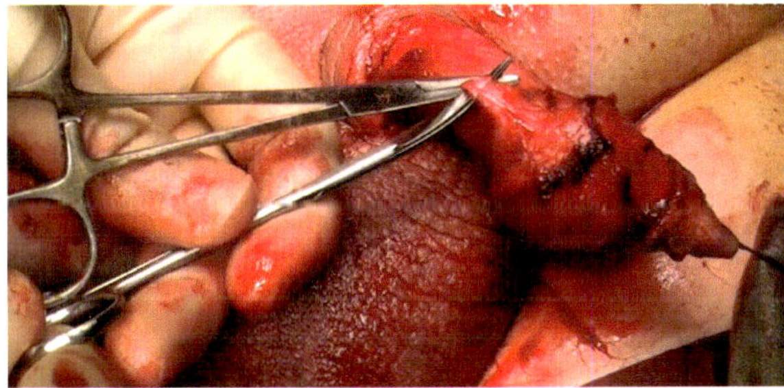

Fig. 10.13 Dissection under Buck's fascia with identification of the neurovascular bundle

analogous to dissection over Buck's fascia, except for the STSG which is placed directly to the tunica albuginea. Post-operative dressing and management is identical to glans resurfacing.

Glansectomy offers good oncological and functional results. Most patients maintain sexual penile functions, except for glans sensitivity reduction [25, 26]. However, a lack of good data on functional and sexual outcomes exists, and these claims are based on our experience. Most common complications are partial or complete graft loss, meatal stenosis, and infection. In a series of 145 patients, partial graft loss and total graft loss were 20% and 3.4%, respectively [22]. Local recurrence rates are between 4%–9.3%, depending on tumour stage [22, 27].

Distal Urethroplasty with Buccal Mucosa Graft (BMG): Harvesting, Application and Wound Care

If a tumour involves the glans and the distal penile urethra, partial glansectomy and distal urethrectomy can be performed. Surgical urethral excision is followed by urethroplasty, which can be done in a one- or two-staged procedure. The extent of urethral excision affects the reconstructive treatment options, which include formation of an heterotopic neomeatus or construction of an orthotopic neourethra with BMG [14]. Buccal mucosa grafts have emerged as an attractive graft choice due to the tissue's biologic characteristics. First, buccal mucosa is accessible and easy to harvest. Second, the donor site is concealed and therefore potential scar tissue is not visible. Third, buccal mucosa has a thick epithelium and a thin, highly vascularized lamina propria, which enhances graft take rates [28].

Buccal Mucosa Graft Harvesting and Wound Care of Donor Site

Mouth cleaning with an oral disinfectant can be started preoperative and continued till 3 days post-operative [29]. The patient is placed in supine position and nasotracheal intubation is preferred, with the throat packed with gauzes. The cheek is prepared and cleaned. A retractor is placed into the mouth to stretch the buccal mucosa [28]. Afterwards the desired graft size is measured and indicated with a pen. Care should be taken to avoid Stensen's duct, with a margin of 1.5 cm [30]. Stay sutures are placed along the graft edges to stretch the buccal mucosa (Fig. 10.14). The buccal donor site is infiltrated with lidocaine hydrochloride 1% with epinephrine

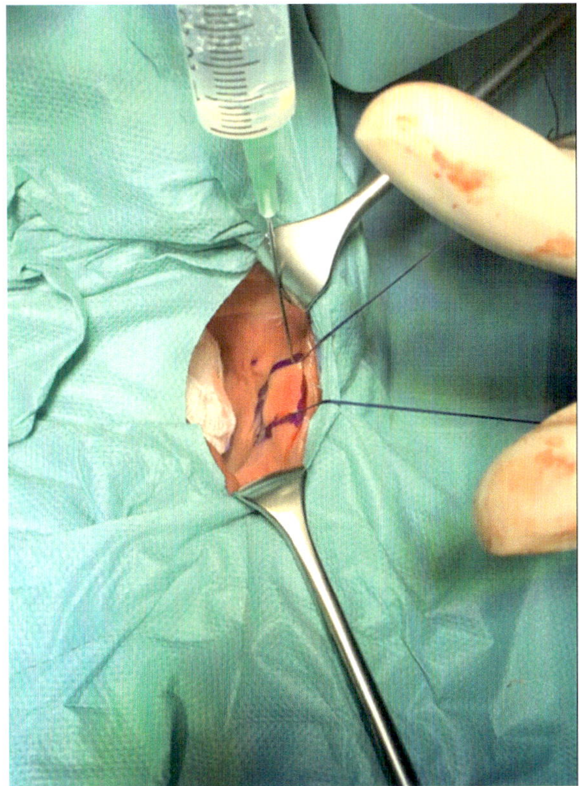

Fig. 10.14 The buccal mucosa graft is indicated and stretched with stay sutures. Hydrodissection is achieved by means of infiltration with Lidocaine hydrochloride 1% and with epinephrine 1:100,000 to enhance haemostasis of the donor site

1:100,000 to enhance haemostasis and to achieve hydrodissection (Fig. 10.14). Afterwards the marked graft is dissected and removed, leaving the muscular fibres intact [30]. The donor site is closed with a continuous suture and preferably without tension. The graft is carefully defatted and prepared for reconstruction of the glans cleft (Fig. 10.15).

Most common complications of buccal graft harvesting are bleeding of donor site, swelling, numbness due to the stitches, and infection [30]. One day postoperative, a liquid diet can be consumed, which can be augmented to a soft diet and then a regular diet afterwards. All patients confirmed eating normally one month after surgery [30].

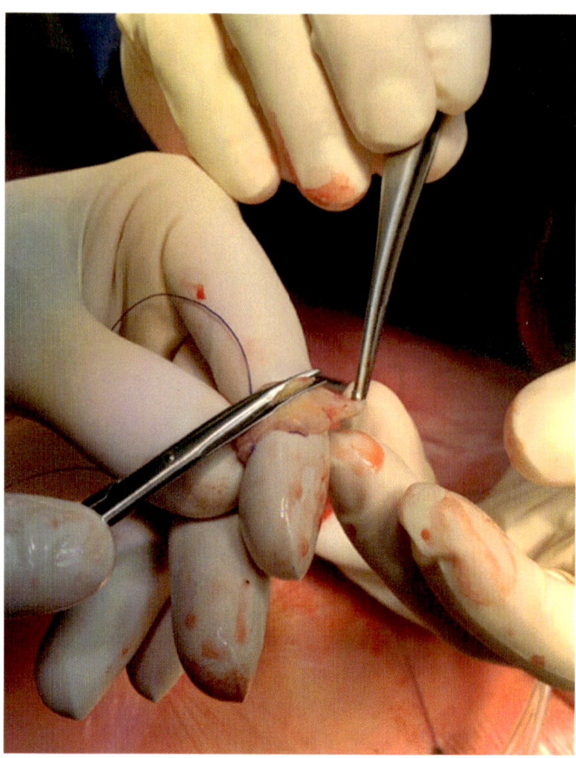

Fig. 10.15 The BMG is carefully defatted and prepared

Application of the Graft

This technique can be offered for pT1 or pT2 lesions with invasion in the urethra. Wide excision of the ventral glans and distal urethra is performed to excise the localized lesion and preserve a part of the native glans. The diseased urothelium is excised ventrally and the glans cleft is deepened [31]. The graft is sewn into the glans cleft with the mucosal part facing the lumen, this forms the neourethral plate (Fig. 10.16) [28]. Afterwards, a tie-over dressing is applied to gently compress the graft. During the first-time procedure, the glans is not closed to optimize graft healing. In addition, the glans cleft is left open to enable oncological control and to allow early diagnosis of tumour recurrence. During the second time, the glans can be closed. However, in our experience most patients do not desire a second operation, as the lesion is located ventrally and not visible most of the time (Fig. 10.17).

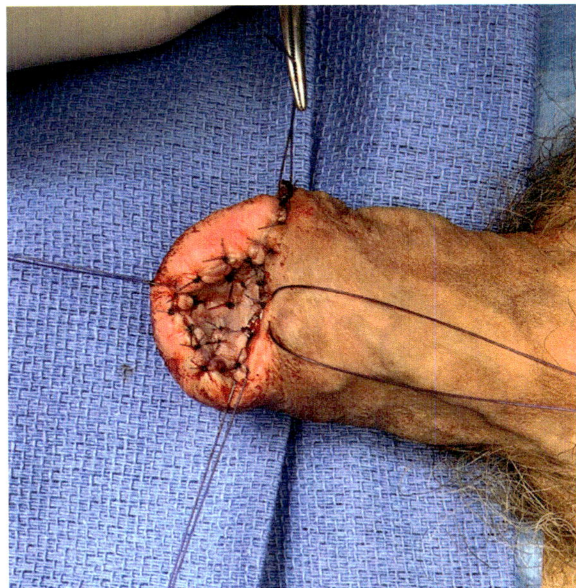

Fig. 10.16 The graft is sewn into the glans cleft with the mucosal part facing the lumen

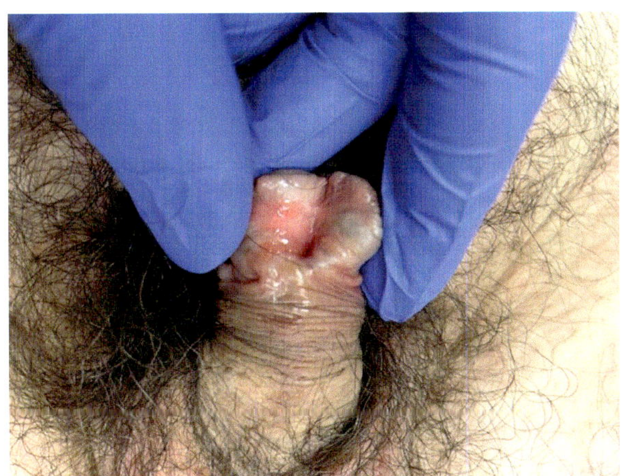

Fig. 10.17 Appearance of a buccal mucosa inlay without closure, one-year post-operative

Partial Penectomy

In cases of extensive disease, with invasion into the corpora cavernosa (cT3) a partial penectomy is advised. Care must be taken to leave a penile stump of sufficient length, considering the patient's genitourinary function including micturition and sexual activity [14]. If a significant portion of the penis must be removed, a total penectomy with perineal urethrostomy may be the preferred treatment to avoid the urinary stream passing over the scrotum during voiding. The primary objective of a partial penectomy is cancer control. The secondary objective is the ability to void in the standing position and to preserve sexual function as much as possible [7].

Surgical Technique

This technique is usually performed under general anaesthetic and local penile block. Broad spectrum antibiotics are administered preoperatively. A circumferential incision is made in the penile skin proximal to the tumour. Although there is no straight consensus on resection margins, there is a paradigm shift towards smaller margins to improve functional and aesthetic results. Although, in the tumours amenable to partial penectomy, broader margins should be considered as these are high risk lesions in which local recurrence is predictive for disease specific survival [11, 32]. The dissection continues until Buck's fascia is reached and the dorsal neurovascular bundle is identified. Afterwards the dorsal neurovascular bundle is ligated [7]. After applying a tourniquet, the corpus cavernosum is transected, thereby preserving the corpus spongiosum. The urethra is dissected from the corpus spongiosum and transected, thereby preserving a urethral stump of 1 to 1.5 cm [33]. The corpus cavernosum is oversewn with 2.0 or 3.0 absorbable sutures [7, 33]. Afterwards the urethral stump is spatulated dorsally and brought through the ventral penile skin. The spatulated urethra is fixed to the penile shaft skin [4]. Finally, the penile shaft skin is sutured using 3.0 or 4.0 absorbable sutures. During this technique, the tourniquet can intermittently be released to identify bleeding vessels and perform a good haemostasis.

This technique provides less attractive aesthetic results because of the appearance of the ventrally located urethra, causing psychological morbidity. Moreover, most common complication is meatal stenosis. Several alternative techniques have been described.

A first example is the formation of a neoglans. The distal end of the corpus cavernosum can be used to create a neoglans as described in the glansectomy surgical technique. In this case, a STSG from the thigh is harvested to cover the distal corporal tips. This technique provides better cosmetical results and is indicated in men who have sufficient remaining penile length after partial penectomy to construct a neoglans.

Another variation is a partial penectomy with urethral centralization which allows a more centralized urethral meatus. This technique is called urethral centralization after partial penectomy (UCAPP), first described by Kranz. et al. [34]. UCAPP aims to reduce the psychological morbidity and to optimize the aesthetic appearance [4, 7]. Here the urethra is dissected from the tunica albuginea. Afterwards a small incision is made in the ventral septum pectiniform, which splits both corpora cavernosa [34]. The urethra is mobilized and sutured at a 12 o' clock position directly to the tunica albuginea of the corpora cavernosa. The exposed corpora cavernosa are covered by the outer fascia of the corpus spongiosum.

The tunica albuginea of each corpora cavernosa is sutured together at the 6 o' clock position, which allows the formation of a urethrostomy at the distal end of the corpora [4, 7]. Both corpora surround the entire urethra which provides a good haemostasis. The penile shaft skin is sutured to the tunica albuginea of both corpora, thereby leaving the distal corporal heads exposed. Afterwards a neoglans is created, using a STSG as described before.

Post-operative a dressing is sutured to the neoglans, and a catheter is placed. These are removed 7–10 days post-operative [4, 34]. Broad spectrum antibiotics are continued for 5 days [34]. There is a lack of data, specified on local recurrence after partial penectomy. Horenblas et al. described a. local recurrence rate of 8% for the whole amputation group (partial + total penectomy) [35]. Furthermore, recurrence rate is depending on tumour stage with local recurrence rates of 18 to 20% in T2 and T3 tumours [6].

Total Penectomy + Perineal Urethrostomy

A total penectomy is indicated for locally advanced disease (pT4), when negative surgical margins cannot be achieved through a partial penectomy or when the remaining penile stump is insufficient to obtain a good genitourinary function [33]. After the excision of the penis, a perineal urethrostomy is created, which requires men sitting down to void [4]. In second time, a phallic reconstruction can be considered. Many advanced penile cancers present with a secondary infection, therefore broad-spectrum antibiotics are administered preoperatively.

Surgical Technique

This technique is performed under general anaesthetic. Broad spectrum antibiotics are administered preoperatively. The patient is placed in lithotomy position and a rhombic incision is marked around the penis. Dissection through the skin is performed and the penis is mobilized proximally. Afterwards the suspensory ligament is divided, and dissection continues until the neurovascular bundle is reached and ligated.

An inverted Y-incision is made in the perineum, which will form the urinary outlet. The bulb penis is dissected with preservation of the urethra proximal. Afterwards the proximal crura cavernosa are dissected of the pubic bone. The urethra is transected, brought through the inverted Y-incision, and sutured to the perineum. Care must be taken that the urethra is fixed to the perineum without angulation and with wide ventral spatulation [14].

Post-operative a catheter is placed into the neomeatus and the urethrostomy is covered in a paraffin dressing. The urethral catheter can be removed 5–7 days post-operative. Stenosis of the perineal urethrostomy is a possible and may require future revision surgery [4, 36].

Penile Reconstruction and Phalloplasty

Penile reconstruction or phalloplasty is typically reserved for situations when all other options for reconstruction have failed or are inappropriate. Commonly, this situation arises following total penectomy or where the functional penile length is inadequate for the man to void while standing or to have sexual intercourse.

Phalloplasty was first pioneered by N Bogoraz in 1936 using a tube pedicled abdominal graft and transplanted cartilage as a phallic stiffener [37]. The first patient had suffered traumatic penile amputation but a subsequent case series of 16 men including several men post-penectomy for penile cancer was published 1939. Penile reconstruction is complex and requires an understanding of the relevant anatomy and surgical techniques including microsurgical skills. Men should be referred to a tertiary centre with the necessary expertise but even then, experience can be limited. Only one out of 316 men in a large study reporting the outcomes of phalloplasty had penile cancer [38]. The aim of the following section is to briefly summarise the technical concepts and surgical considerations for phalloplasty in this challenging cohort.

Goals of Surgery

Phalloplasty aims to construct a neophallus following penectomy using a local or distant tissue flap. Distant flaps are transferred as a free flap using microsurgical techniques or as a pedicled flap while maintaining its own blood supply. Currently, the most common flap used is the radial artery forearm free (RFF) flap. Other alternatives include the anterolateral thigh (ALT) flap, musculocutaneous latissimus dorsi (MLD) flap and suprapubic flap [39].

The ideal neophallus should be aesthetically pleasing and sensate (to both erogenous and tactile stimulus) while allowing voiding when standing and sexual intercourse. The ideal technique should achieve these goals in a single operation with minimal donor site morbidity. Disappointingly, no current technique satisfies all the above requirements [39].

Surgical Technique

Penile reconstruction is generally performed over 2–3 stages depending on centre. The first stage involves neophallus creation with integrated urethra followed by microvascular transfer to the recipient site. A glans is then fashioned at the same time or at a later stage (glansplasty). An inflatable penile prosthesis can be inserted after an interval of at least 3 months.

Two surgical teams are usually required for phalloplasty—one team raises the flap while the other prepares the recipient site. The RFF flap is supplied by the radial artery while venous outflow is via the cephalic and basilic veins [40]. The radial artery is anastomosed to the inferior epigastric artery via a groin incision while the veins are anastomosed to branches of the ipsilateral saphenous vein. A "tube within a tube" urethra is integrated in the flap design and an anastomotic urethroplasty to the native urethra is typically performed with a covering suprapubic catheter and urethral stent. Tactile and erogenous sensation in almost 90% of patients is achieved by neurorrhaphy between the lateral antebrachial cutaneous nerves of the forearm with the dorsal penile nerves [40].

Alternatively, an ALT flap may be preferred for a more hidden donor site. The flap is supplied by perforators originating from the lateral circumflex femoral artery with sensation from the lateral femoral cutaneous nerve [41]. The MLD flap tends

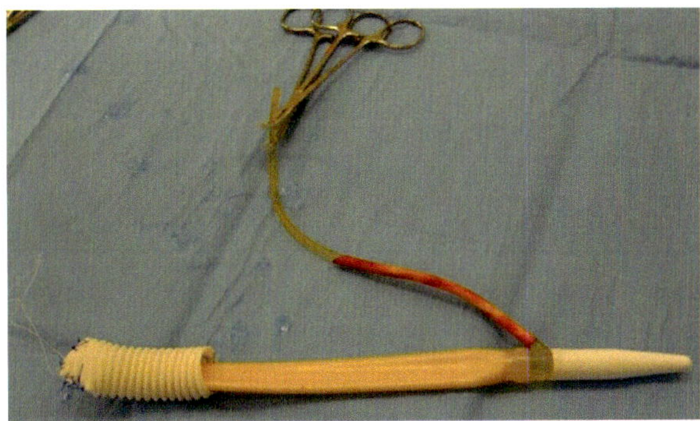

Fig. 10.18 Single cylinder device prepared with Dacron cap in place

to be insensate and is supplied by the thoracodorsal neurovascular bundle. Another advantage of the MLD flap is that the urethra is not integrated into the flap design and therefore may have a poorer blood supply.

Inserting an erectile device is challenging given the lack or loss of typical anatomical landmarks. A rear tip extender or malleable penile prosthesis can be placed in the crus of the penis (if preserved) at the time of phalloplasty to help identify the structures during subsequent penile prosthesis insertion. A penoscrotal incision is typically used and dilatation of the cylinder space within the neophallus is performed to size 18 Hegar [42]. The device is prepared as routine, but a polyethylene terephthalate (Dacron) cap is sutured to the cylinder tip to prevent migration within the neophallus (Fig. 10.18). The device is kept partially inflated for a week to allow a capsule to form.

Specific Considerations Following Penectomy

Penile reconstruction in men following partial or total penectomy can be complicated by scarring from previous surgery and the potential loss of structures that would normally be present at the recipient site. Thorough and precise surgical planning is therefore required when considering penile reconstruction in this population. Ideally, the urologist who performed the penectomy should be consulted or their operation report reviewed. This is not always possible, and it is essential that the reconstructive urologist has the experience to manage unexpected intra-operative findings.

Anastomotic variations may be required when structures like the long saphenous vein and dorsal penile nerves are sacrificed in the primary surgery. Alternative venous anastomoses can be performed to the femoral vein, the venae comitantes of the inferior epigastric artery or the dorsal penile vein, if present. Similarly, neurorrhaphy to the ilio-inguinal nerves or genital branch of the genitofemoral nerve may be required instead.

When present, a perineal urethrostomy will need to be reversed and re-routed to the orthotopic position while maximising native urethral length. Our experience suggests that it is rare for a man to decline reversal of his perineal urethrostomy although this would minimise the risk of future urethral complications.

Surgical and Functional Outcomes

There are little published data on phalloplasty following surgical treatment for penile cancer given the rarity of the condition and complexity of reconstruction. Expertise in phalloplasty has been adapted from the field of transmasculine gender affirmation surgery. Only one cross-sectional retrospective study reported the outcomes of penile reconstruction following penile cancer ($n = 15$) in addition to a handful of case reports [40].

Functional and cosmetic outcomes following RFF phalloplasty were excellent after a median (range) follow-up of 20 (1–68) months. All were satisfied with the cosmesis and size of the neophallus (Figs. 10.19 and 10.20) and 90% of men reported sensation. Five out of seven men with a penile prosthesis could engage in

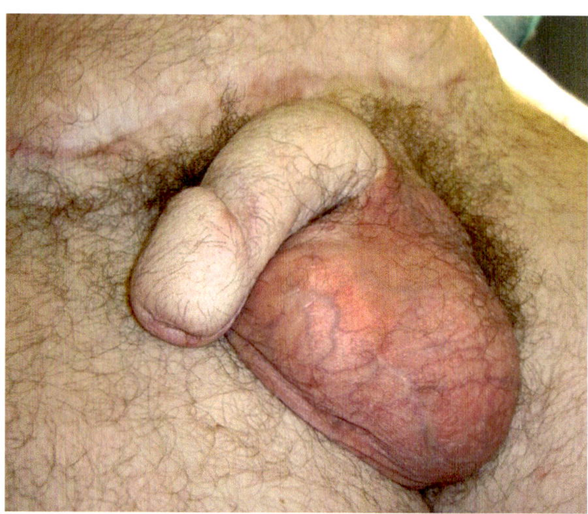

Fig. 10.19 The neophallus deflated

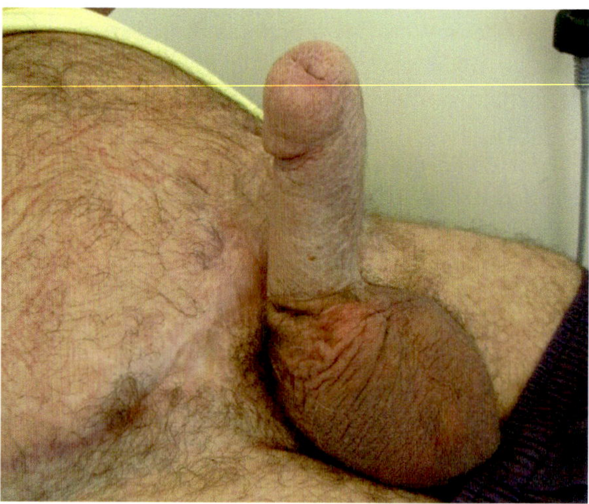

Fig. 10.20 The neophallus inflated

sexual intercourse. Urethral complications (strictures and fistulae) were the most common complication occurring in 47% of men. One man required explant of his penile prosthesis due to infection (14%).

Conclusion

Nowadays, a paradigm shift towards less-invasive organ-sparing surgery in the treatment of localized penile cancer has occurred. Organ-sparing reconstructive techniques improve functional and aesthetic outcomes and consequently minimize psychological and physical morbidity of penile cancer surgery. The extent of tumour invasion will determine between OSS and radical excision treatments. Next to this, a careful patient selection is important, with respect to preoperative pathological risk factors, patient's expectations, and their willingness to maintain strict follow-up.

Key Points

- The surgical treatment of penile cancer has shifted to less-invasive organ-sparing surgery with a reduction in resection margins.
- The aim of organ-sparing reconstructive techniques is to improve functional and aesthetic outcomes and to minimize psychological and physical morbidity.
- A careful patient selection, with respect to preoperative clinical staging and patient's characteristics, is crucial in organ-sparing treatment.
- Patients must be compliant to strict surveillance protocols, because of the higher risk of local recurrence after organ-sparing surgery.

Revision Questions

Multiple Choice Questions

1. A 40 years old patient presents with a red superficial lesion confined to the prepuce. What is the best treatment in this young patient?
   A. Partial glansectomy
   B. Wide local excision
   C. Total glansectomy with STSG
   D. Circumcision
2. In buccal mucosa graft harvesting, care should be taken to avoid which structure:
   A. Wharton's duct
   B. Sublingual duct
   C. Stensen's duct
   D. Facial nerve

3. A 55 year old patient underwent 4 years ago a glansectomy because of a pT2 penile SCC. The first 2 years after surgery and in the third and fourth year, he had 3-monthly and 6-monthly examinations, respectively, without recurrence of tumour lesions. Currently, he represents with a fixed nodule on the dorsal side of the penis perimeatal. However, the clinical examination is not clear and cannot differentiate between a tumour recurrence inside the corpora or scar tissue after primary surgery. Which examination can you use?
   A. Penile ultrasound
   B. MRI in erect state
   C. PET-CT
   D. RX

Viva Cases

Case 1

A Male patient, 71 years old presents to you in clinic.

Medical history:

He presents with a 1-year difficulty with retracting the prepuce over the glans penis (phimosis). The patient has noticed since more than 2 months a fixed palpable red lesion on the glans penis. He has no other complaints with normal Miction and no other lesions on his body.

Past Medical History:

- 2018: intermittent claudication left leg
- 2020: triple coronary artery bypass grafting
- chronic obstructive pulmonary disease

Current Medications:

- Acidum acetylsalicylicum 80 mg
- Atorvastatin 80 mg
- Omeprazole 40 mg

Social History:

- Smoking History of ±50 pack years
- Alcohol: 4 units/week
- No medical history of sexually transmitted infections.

Clinical examination:

- Phimosis
- Red lesion on glans penis, dorsal of the meatus. This lesion is fixed and has an ulcerated aspect.
- Lymph nodes: not palpable

A subsequent excision biopsy was done and showed an invasive lesion in the corpus spongiosum, without invasion into the corpus cavernosum: pathological staging pT2.

A. Which surgical treatment should you advice?

Case 2
A 64-year-old male patient presents to you.

The patient presents with a big nodule on the glans. Now for 2 months he has noted sometimes blood on the lesion and besides he mentions that the lesion is painful.

Miction is more difficult compared to last year. He suffers frequency, intermittency, and spraying. He has no other lesions on his body.

Past Medical History:

- Previous appendectomy

Current Medications:

- Nil

Social History

- Cigarettes: Nil
- Alcohol: 2 units/week
- No medical history of sexually transmitted infections.

Clinical examination:

- There is a big nodule ventrally on the glans penis, with a fixed and firm aspect and palpable in the distal urethra
- Clinical no lesions palpable in the corpora cavernosa.
- Lymph nodes: not palpable.

The patient subsequently underwent a total glansectomy, although postoperative the pathological report describes positive section margins. Bilateral dynamic sentinel node biopsy was negative.

A. Which treatment should you advice regarding this medical history and in case of positive sections margins after total glansectomy?

Answers

Multiple Choice Questions

1. **D.** Circumcision offers a good and effective treatment option for lesions which are confined to the prepuce.
2. **C.** Stensen's duct, which is the major salivary duct of the parotid gland is an important anatomical consideration when conducting harvesting.
3. **B.** An MRI in an erect state can differentiate about invasion into the corpora.

Viva Cases

Case 1

A. A glansectomy is the best organ-sparing treatment in which you can maintain penile function as much as oncologically possible. In this case a glansectomy with STSG should be avoided. A STSG in a patient with vascular disease has a significantly bigger chance to fail or infect.

When you do not have any suspicion for corporal tip involvement, dissection over Buck's fascia is preferable to protect the dorsal neurovascular bundle. M.

Make sure you discuss with the patient his preferences and expectances in advance. A partial penectomy should also be an appropriate treatment, however more debilitating.

Case 2

A. A partial penectomy might have been a better option. When clinically questionable, a biopsy might have been done before surgery. In this case, tumour was invading the corpora cavernosa so a partial penectomy must be considered. After partial penectomy, pathological staging was pT3NO with negative section margins.

Test your learning and check your understanding of this book's contents: use the "Springer Nature Flashcards" app to access questions using ▸ https://sn.pub/1r7Om8. To use the app, please follow the instructions in chapter 1.

References

1. Thomas A, Necchi A, Muneer A, Tobias-Machado M, Tran ATH, Van Rompuy A-S, et al. Penile cancer. Nat Rev Dis Primers. 2021;7:1.
2. Amin MBES, Greene FL, et al. AJCC cancer staging manual. 8th ed. NewYork: Springer; 2017.
3. Alnajjar HM, Randhawa K, Muneer A. Localized disease: types of reconstruction/plastic surgery techniques after glans resurfacing/glansectomy/partial/total penectomy. Curr Opin Urol. 2020;30(2):213–7.

4. Pang KH, Alnajjar HM, Muneer A. Management of Primary Penile Tumours: partial and Total penectomy. Penile Carcinoma. 2021:75–84.
5. Skrodzka M, Ayres B, Watkin N. Penile-sparing surgical and non-surgical approaches. Penile Carcinoma. 2021:59–73.
6. Raskin Y, Vanthoor J, Milenkovic U, Muneer A, Albersen M. Organ-sparing surgical and non-surgical modalities in primary penile cancer treatment. Curr Opin Urol. 2019;29(2):156–64.
7. Horenblas S, Malone P, Muneer A. Surgical treatment of penile cancer. 2013. 134–50.
8. Leijte JA, Kirrander P, Antonini N, Windahl T, Horenblas S. Recurrence patterns of squamous cell carcinoma of the penis: recommendations for follow-up based on a two-Centre analysis of 700 patients. Eur Urol. 2008;54(1):161–8.
9. Philippou P, Shabbir M, Malone P, Nigam R, Muneer A, Ralph DJ, et al. Conservative surgery for squamous cell carcinoma of the penis: resection margins and long-term oncological control. J Urol. 2012;188(3):803–8.
10. Sri D, Sujenthiran A, Lam W, Minter J, Tinwell BE, Corbishley CM, et al. A study into the association between local recurrence rates and surgical resection margins in organ-sparing surgery for penile squamous cell cancer. BJU Int. 2018;122(4):576–82.
11. Roussel E, Peeters E, Vanthoor J, Bozzini G, Muneer A, Ayres B, et al. Predictors of local recurrence and its impact on survival after glansectomy for penile cancer: time to challenge the dogma? BJU Int. 2021;127(5):606–13.
12. O.W. Hakenberg (Chair) EC, S. Minhas, A. Necchi CP, N. Watkin (Vice-chair). Guidelines on penile cancer 2018 [Available from: https://uroweb.org/wp-content/uploads/EAU-Guidelines-Penile-Cancer-2018.pdf].
13. Thomas W. Flaig PES, et al. National Comprehensive Cancer Network. Guidelines on penile cancer 2021 [Available from: https://www.nccn.org/professionals/physician_gls/pdf/penile.pdf].
14. Burnett AL. Penile preserving and reconstructive surgery in the management of penile cancer. Nat Rev Urol. 2016;13(5):249–57.
15. Bronselaer GA, Schober JM, Meyer-Bahlburg HFL, T'Sjoen G, Vlietinck R, Hoebeke PB. Male circumcision decreases penile sensitivity as measured in a large cohort. BJU Int. 2013;111(5):820–7.
16. Cakir OO, Schifano N, Venturino L, Pozzi E, Castiglione F, Alnajjar HM, et al. Surgical technique and outcomes following coronal-sparing glans resurfacing for benign and malignant penile lesions. Int J Impot Res. 2021;
17. Shabbir M, Muneer A, Kalsi J, Shukla CJ, Zacharakis E, Garaffa G, et al. Glans resurfacing for the treatment of carcinoma in situ of the penis: surgical technique and outcomes. Eur Urol. 2011;59(1):142–7.
18. Issa A, Sebro K, Kwok A, Janisch F, Grossmann NC, Lee E, et al. Treatment options and outcomes for men with penile intraepithelial neoplasia: a systematic review. Eur Urol Focus.
19. Pappas A, Katafigiotis I, Waterloos M, Spinoit AF, Ploumidis A. Glans resurfacing with skin graft for penile cancer: a step-by-step video presentation of the technique and review of the literature. Biomed Res Int. 2019;2019:5219048.
20. Malone PR, Thomas JS, Blick C. A tie-over dressing for graft application in distal penectomy and glans resurfacing: the TODGA technique. BJU Int. 2011;107(5):836–40.
21. Hadway P, Corbishley CM, Watkin NA. Total glans resurfacing for premalignant lesions of the penis: initial outcome data. BJU Int. 2006;98(3):532–6.
22. Parnham AS, Albersen M, Sahdev V, Christodoulidou M, Nigam R, Malone P, et al. Glansectomy and Split-thickness skin graft for penile cancer. Eur Urol. 2018;73(2):284–9.
23. Mosahebi A, Woollard ACS. Basic surgical techniques. Atlas of Male Genitourethral Surgery. 2014:14–24.
24. Austoni E, Fenice O, Kartalas Goumas Y, Colombo F, Mantovani F, Pisani E. New trends in the surgical treatment of penile carcinoma. Arch Ital Urol Androl. 1996;68(3):163–8.
25. Gulino G, Sasso F, Falabella R, Bassi PF. Distal urethral reconstruction of the glans for penile carcinoma: results of a novel technique at 1-year of followup. J Urol. 2007;178(3 Pt 1):941–4.

26. Morelli G, Pagni R, Mariani C, Campo G, Menchini-Fabris F, Minervini R, et al. Glansectomy with split-thickness skin graft for the treatment of penile carcinoma. Int J Impot Res. 2009;21(5):311–4.
27. Smith Y, Hadway P, Biedrzycki O, Perry MJ, Corbishley C, Watkin NA. Reconstructive surgery for invasive squamous carcinoma of the glans penis. Eur Urol. 2007;52(4):1179–85.
28. Kane CJ, Tarman GJ, Summerton DJ, Buchmann CE, Ward JF, O'Reilly KJ, et al. Multi-institutional experience with buccal mucosa onlay urethroplasty for bulbar urethral reconstruction. J Urol. 2002;167(3):1314–7.
29. Aldaqadossi H, El Gamal S, El-Nadey M, El Gamal O, Radwan M, Gaber M. Dorsal onlay (Barbagli technique) versus dorsal inlay (Asopa technique) buccal mucosal graft urethroplasty for anterior urethral stricture: a prospective randomized study. Int J Urol. 2014;21(2):185–8.
30. Barbagli G, Vallasciani S, Romano G, Fabbri F, Guazzoni G, Lazzeri M. Morbidity of oral mucosa graft harvesting from a single cheek. Eur Urol. 2010;58(1):33–41.
31. Andrich D, Mundy T. In: Atlas of male genitourethral surgery: the illustrated guide. ed: Muneer A. 2013. p. 117–33.
32. Djajadiningrat RS, EvW WM, van Rhijn BWG, Bex A, van der Poel HG, Horenblas S. Penile sparing surgery for penile cancer—does it affect survival? J Urol. 2014.
33. Gonzalgo M, Parekh D. Partial penectomy. In: Hinman's Atlas of Urologic Surgery. 2012. p. 113–8. https://doi.org/10.1016/B978-1-4160-4210-5.00027-X.
34. Kranz J, Parnham A, Albersen M, Sahdev V, Ziada M, Nigam R, et al. Zentralisierung der Harnröhre und Pseudoglansbildung nach partieller Penektomie. Urologe. 2017;56(10):1293–7.
35. Horenblas S. Squamous cell carcinoma of the penis. II. Treatment of the primary tumor. J Urol. 1992;
36. De Vries HM, Chipollini J, Slongo J, Boyd F, Korkes F, Albersen M, et al. Outcomes of perineal urethrostomy for penile cancer: a 20-year international multicenter experience. Urol Oncol. 2021;39(8):500.e9-.e13
37. Schultheiss D, Gabouev AI, Jonas U. Nikolaj A. Bogoraz: Pioneer of phalloplasty and penile implant surgery. J Sex Med. 2005;2(1):139–46.
38. Doornaert M, Hoebeke P, Ceulemans P, T'Sjoen G, Heylens G, Monstrey S. Penile reconstruction with the radial forearm flap: an update. Handchir Mikrochir Plast Chir. 2011;43(4):208–14.
39. Lee WG, Christopher N, Ralph DJ. Penile reconstruction and the role of surgery in gender dysphoria. Eur Urol Focus. 2019;5(3):337–9.
40. Garaffa G, Raheem AA, Christopher NA, Ralph DJ. Total phallic reconstruction after penile amputation for carcinoma. BJU Int. 2009;104(6):852–6.
41. Lee GK, Lim AF, Bird ET. A novel single-flap technique for total penile reconstruction: the pedicled anterolateral thigh flap. Plast Reconstr Surg. 2009;124(1):163–6.
42. Lee WG CA, Ralph DJ. IPP in neophallus. In Mulcahy J MI, Garcia E and Salamanca J, editor 2020. 213–31 p.

Late Effects of Penile Cancer

11

Clare Akers, Stanley Tang, Oliver Brunckhorst, and Matthew Rewhorn

Learning Objectives

After reading this chapter you will be able to:

- Describe common urinary and sexual changes that can occur following previous management for penile cancer
- Explain the sequela and classification of lymphoedema following penile cancer treatment
- Discuss conservative and surgical management options for patients with late effects of penile cancer
- Recognise the physical and psychosocial implications for patients experiencing these changes after diagnosis.

Introduction

Conventional cancer therapies, including radiotherapy and inguinal lymphadenectomy, have made significant improvements in the treatment outcomes and prognosis of penile cancer patients. Nevertheless, despite various advances in techniques to improve outcomes and decrease morbidity, these interventions can leave patients

C. Akers · S. Tang
Department of Urology, University College London Hospital, London, UK

O. Brunckhorst
MRC Centre for Transplantation, Guy's Hospital Campus, King's College London, King's Health Partners, London, UK

M. Rewhorn (✉)
Department of Urology, NHS Greater Glasgow & Clyde, Glasgow, UK
e-mail: m.rewhorn@nhs.net

O. Brunckhorst et al. (eds.), *Penile Cancer – A Practical Guide*, Management of Urology, https://doi.org/10.1007/978-3-031-32681-3_11

with significant life changing complications, that can have major functional, psychological, and cosmetic side effects. These side effects not only burden patients and affect their quality of life (QoL) but also that of their partner [1, 2]. Long term side effects include changes to urinary and sexual function as well as genital and lower limb lymphoedema. Often these side effects are underdiagnosed and undertreated adding to patient frustration with chronic disease.

Urinary Changes

Following surgery most men remain continent as both bladder neck and sphincter remain competent. The external length of the penis will have changed however. People who have undergone glansectomy or partial penectomy should still be able to stand to micturate but may have problems including spraying of urine or poor flow if they develop stenosis at their neourethra (Fig. 11.1). Patients who have undergone a more radical procedure such as total penectomy and formation of a perineal urethrostomy should be consented for their need to sit to urinate. During follow up of such patients if they describe voiding difficulty, examination, which

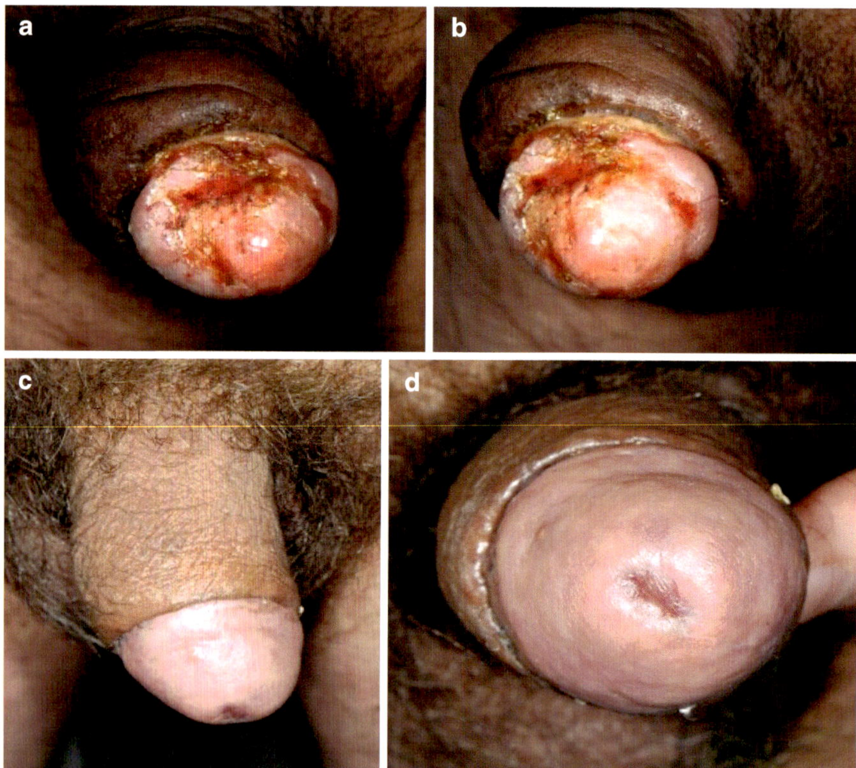

Fig. 11.1 (**a**, **b**) Meatal Stenosis with Lichen Sclerosus and Penile Carcinoma in Situ (**c**, **d**) Meatal Stenosis After Glans Resurfacing

may include cystoscopy, should be performed to look for urethral strictures or stenosis of the urethra.

Some patients following treatment desire reconstructive surgery for voiding and sexual function and these reconstructive surgeries including phalloplasty have been described earlier in the book.

Sexual Changes

Maintaining adequate sexual function is an important consideration for patients undergoing surgical intervention for penile cancer [3]. Operative intervention for penile cancer will invariably have a negative effect on sexual function. This is most commonly due to physiological and psychological factors. Studies comparing sexual function pre- and post-operatively using questionnaires such as the International Index of Erectile Dysfunction (IIEF) show a reduction in overall satisfaction, although this is dependent on the procedure, with more radical procedures leading to lower sexual satisfaction [4]. Wide local excision or more recently, glans resurfacing, have encouraging satisfaction rates [5].

Psychosexual issues frequently contribute to overall sexual dissatisfaction after penile cancer treatment. Glansectomy and partial penectomy penile cosmesis, which can alter patient perception of self and body image [6]. Pre-operative expectation management is important in that respect. Reduction in penis size has been reported as a barrier to sexual satisfaction post-operatively, with a median penile length in some studies quoted as 4 cm in flaccid state [7].

There is a risk of reduced sexual sensation after glansectomy or partial penectomy. Despite this, over half of patients can achieve erection sufficient for intercourse [7]. Factors increasing the likelihood of erectile dysfunction include increasing age, shorter penile shaft length and clinically positive lymph nodes [3].

Lymphoedema

The lymphatic drainage from the penis and scrotum is primarily to the inguinal lymph nodes, in turn draining into the pelvic lymph nodes. Disruption to these channels by either surgical intervention or radiotherapy treatment can lead to lymphoedema within the tissue.

Lymphoedema describes a progressive pathologic condition of the lymphatic system in which there is interstitial accumulation of protein-rich fluid and subsequent inflammation, adipose tissue hypertrophy, and fibrosis [8]. Under normal circumstances the efflux from capillaries that accumulates in the interstitium is reabsorbed primarily by venous capillaries (90%) whilst the remainder is transported via the lymphatics as lymph. Disruption of this normal lymphatic system reduces the capacity of re-absorption and fluid accumulates leading to the characteristic swelling of lymphoedema [8]. Moreover, lymphatics normally assist in the transport of degraded interstitial proteins to allow them to be reabsorbed into the circulation, but absence of lymphatics leads to higher interstitial protein concentration, increasing colloid osmotic pressure further driving fluid into the interstitial space [9]. Recurrent cellulitis can further contribute to loss of elasticity, hyperplasia of collagenous connective tissue and ultimately fibrosis which compounds tissue dysfunction [10]. The clinical manifestation of this results in skin disorders including hyperkeratosis, dermal thickening, hyperpigmentation, increased skin folds, warty overgrowths, and rarely malignant transformation.

The classification of lymphoedema can either be primary or secondary [11]. Primary lymphoedema is either congenital or intrinsic dysfunction of lymphatics and may be caused by the obstruction, malformation, or underdevelopment (hypoplasia) of various lymphatic vessels [12]. Secondary lymphoedema however, which occurs after the diagnosis of advanced penile cancer or post-treatment in penile cancer, occurs due to destruction of lymphatics due to the disease or iatrogenic process.

Diagnosis of genital lymphoedema is made through the patient's history and clinical examination findings. Genital lymphoedema (Fig. 11.2) is an uncommon and disabling disease that manifests as enlargement of the genital region due to impaired lymphatic drainage through inguinal lymph nodes [13]. The penis drains in a systematic fashion to the inguinal lymph nodes then to the pelvic lymph nodes and surgery or radiotherapy leads to lymphatic destruction and retention of lymph fluid within the subcutaneous tissue of the genitals and lower limb. This can cause chronic irritation, prevent adequate hygiene measures being performed and impair mobility and ambulation. Moreover, severe forms can lead to penile burying and voiding dysfunction with subsequent secondary infection or prevent sexual intercourse [14, 15]. A severe form of lymphoedema, lymphangitis circumscripta leads to persistent serous discharge and can be debilitating for patients. Repeated cellulitis and lymphangiosarcoma are potential life-threatening sequelae for patients.

The best way to treat side effects is to minimise the morbidity in the first place and has involved development of surgical techniques to minimise lymphatic and nodal disturbance in the first place. Modified inguinal lymph node dissection has been

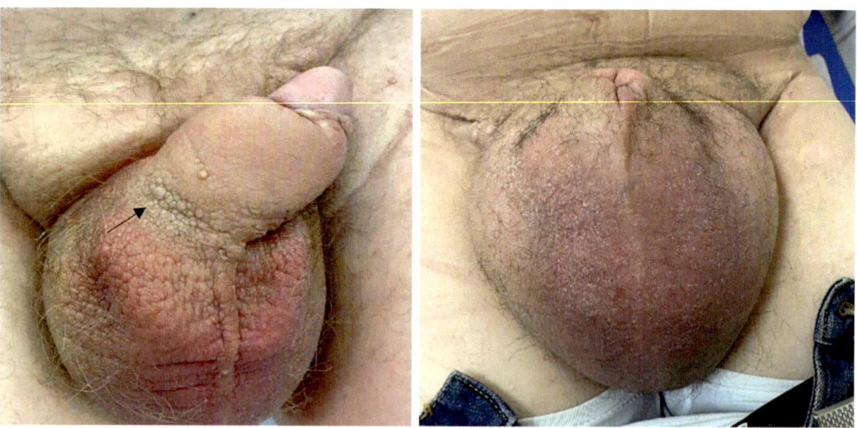

Fig. 11.2 Penile lymphoedema with lymphangioma circumscriptum (arrow) (Images courtesy of Mr. Hussain Alnajjar, UCLH)

largely superseded by dynamic sentinel node biopsy. Positive histology, however, still necessitates the need for completion radical inguinal lymph node dissection. This morbid procedure has risks including infection, bleeding, skin, necrosis, deep vein thrombosis, pulmonary emboli and lymphoedema. Morbidity of conventional inguinal lymphadenectomy has been reported to be as high as 30–50% [16, 17].

Most units in the UK have dedicated lymphoedema nurse specialists that will institute Decongestive Lymphatic Therapy (DLT). These treatment strategies include skin care to reduce infection, exercise to assist lymphatic drainage and reduce adipose tissue, and compression techniques to reduce swelling. Compression hosiery or bandaging can be used in combination with specialised massage called manual lymphatic drainage. If the lymphoedema is severe and not responding to these conservative approaches, then there are more aggressive lines of treatment including liposuction and surgery. Many surgical options have been described in treating lymphoedema including scrotal flaps, skin grafting, tissue debulking or lymphatic restoration.

Surgical treatments should be confined to centres of expertise. Surgical debulking of lymphoedematous tissue of the scrotum whilst maintaining the lateral scrotal flaps allows the testicles to be buried whilst preventing the issue of re-occurrence (Fig. 11.3). The penis can be brought out through a separate incision and grafted [18].

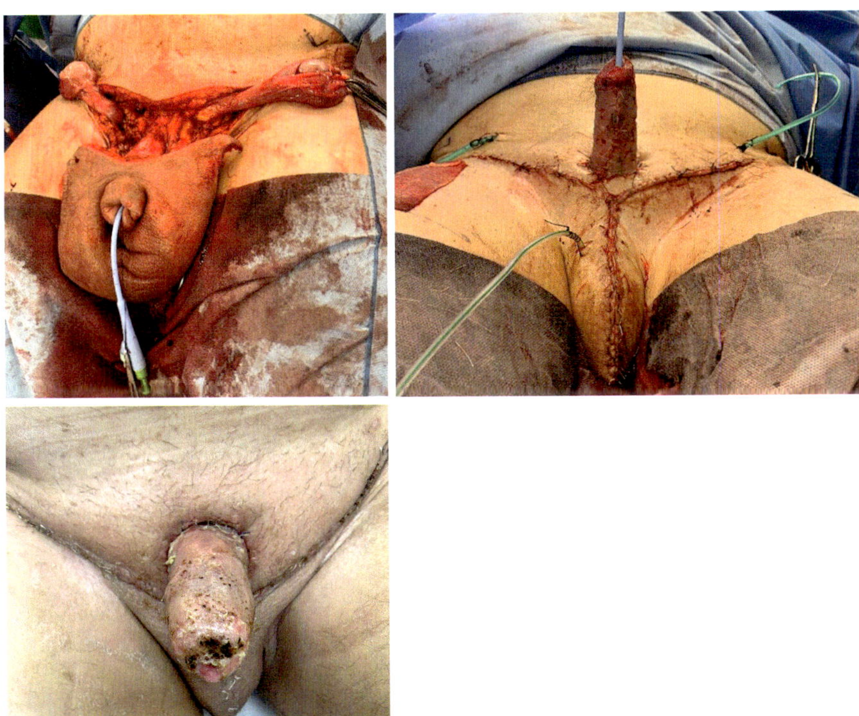

Fig. 11.3 Batman Technique for genital lymphoedema (Images courtesy of Mr. Hussain Alnajjar, UCLH)

Psychosocial Wellbeing in Penile Cancer

There remains a strong focus on the physical sequalae of penile cancer disease, however it is important to also consider the psychosocial wellbeing of patients. Considering the substantial sexual and urinary effects experienced, combined with the role of the penis in men's self-image, it is not surprising to find significant psychosocial late effects in penile cancer.

Defining Psychosocial Wellbeing

Wellbeing is an often broad and poorly defined concept within cancer care. It is however acknowledged to be a multi-dimensional concept with several interacting elements [19]. Mental and social wellbeing are two of these important aspects, possessing a close relationship with the physical health of individuals (Fig. 11.4). Whilst exact components of mental wellbeing are again poorly defined, several elements are found to be repeatedly significant across men's cancer care [20]. Traditionally, many immediately jump to think about mental health disorders such as depression and anxiety when the term is used, and these certainly do have a large role when considering mental wellbeing. However, within cancer care, it is also important to consider other constructs, including the altered perceptions of body image and individual masculinity, self-esteem, and fear of cancer recurrence,

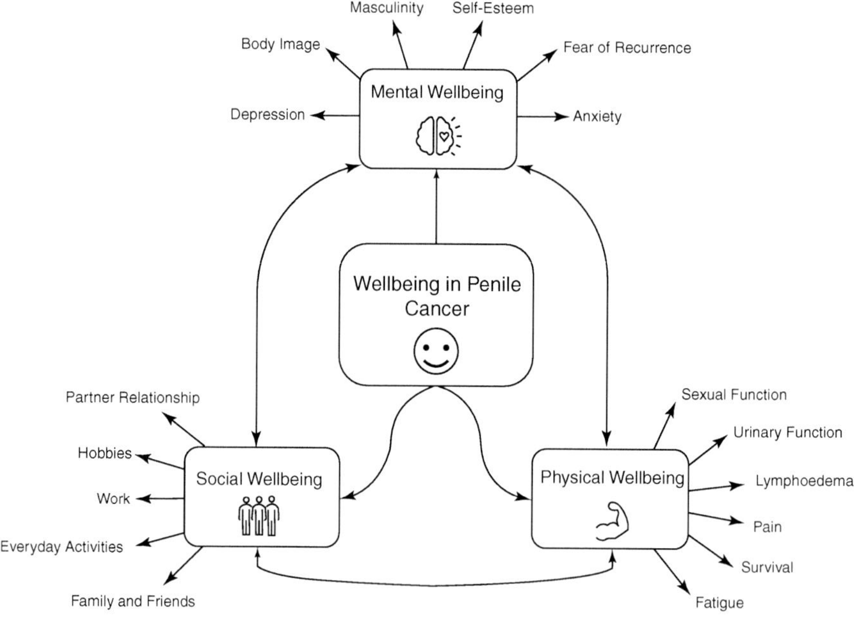

Fig. 11.4 Components of wellbeing in penile cancer

previously labelled as one of the most common unmet needs in cancer [21]. Similarly, considering different components of social wellbeing allows for a broader evaluation of patients. Once again, social wellbeing remains a poorly defined concept, however, important elements to consider include an individual's ability to form meaningful relationships and interactions with others such as partners or significant others, family, friends, work colleagues and the wider society [22]. Additionally, social wellbeing also encompasses the individual's social ability to carry out activities of daily living such as work and hobbies [22, 23].

Psychosocial Impact of Penile Cancer

Due to the relatively rare nature of penile cancer, there is still limited evidence demonstrating the true psychosocial impact of disease on patients. However, the evidence that exists demonstrates the potential severity of symptoms experienced, with some studies estimating over half of individuals experience some psychiatric symptoms with high depressive and anxiety symptoms experienced [24]. This is true particularly after operative treatment with significant anxiety symptoms seen in nearly a third of patients in one study, and a requirement for inpatient psychosocial care in over two thirds of patients [25–28]. When considering other aspects of mental wellbeing, qualitative studies have consistently highlighted the profound impact on masculinity, body image and self-esteem, particularly with more radical surgical treatment options [29–32]. Similarly, fear of cancer recurrence also appears to be a prominent issue for some [29]. These findings are unsurprising considering the penis is an important aspect of men's body image, manhood and sense of identity for many. Similarly, previous research also highlights how relationships are affected post operatively, with the linking factor between many of the issues encountered being subsequent alterations in sexual functioning [31]. This highlights the interlinking nature of many elements across individuals' wellbeing. This is demonstrated through the close association seen between anxiety and depressive symptoms and sexual function after partial penectomy [33]. This close relationship between mental wellbeing and functional and mortality outcomes is also consistently seen amongst other urological malignancies, particularly in male cancers [34]. It is therefore important to consider all elements together during follow up care to ensure better survivorship outcomes for patients.

Improving Psychosocial Outcomes in Penile Cancer

There is unfortunately limited evaluation of penile cancer specific interventions available within the literature. However, general and urological cancer evidence highlights the importance of increased healthcare professionals' awareness of problems that can exist as an important step in ensuring issues are identified, and that appropriate support services are available within existing care pathways [35]. Similarly, patient education on the impact of their condition can have on their mental wellbeing allows patients to remain vigilant, realise what they may experience is not unusual, and can make them more comfortable sharing their experiences with healthcare professionals or with family [35].

It is important that identification of issues occurs during the patient pathway. This can be done informally, or through a more structure approach using patient reported outcome measures (PROMs) or validated psychometric tools (Table 11.1). This allows for early referral to appropriate multidisciplinary support to optimize psychosocial wellbeing outcomes [25]. Whilst it is often outside of the scope of treating clinicians to initiate and undertake complex psychosocial interventions and treatments such as patient education programmes, peer support groups, couples therapy, psychotherapy, or pharmacological psychiatric treatment, it is important to ensure that this expertise is available, with clear referral pathways within the multidisciplinary team. This ensures that true holistic survivorship care can be undertaken to optimise both physical and psychosocial outcomes in penile cancer care.

Key Points

- Secondary lymphoedema is a common manifestation following penile cancer treatment
- Sexual function is frequently impaired following radical surgery
- Surgical techniques have been modified to reduce the risk of lymphoedema
- Considering the psychosocial wellbeing post treatment of penile cancer patients is important for improving survivorship care
- Early recognition and management of all issues discussed are key

Table 11.1 Examples of psychometric tools to evaluate mental wellbeing

Psychometric tool	N. of Items	Properties assessed
Depressive Symptoms		
Center for Epidemiologic Studies Depression Scale (CES-D)	20	Depressed affect, anhedonia, somatic activity, and interpersonal challenges
Hospital Anxiety and Depression Scale – Depression Subscale (HADS-D)	7	Focused on cognitive symptoms of depression rather than somatic symptoms that might reflect the physical condition.
Patient Health Questionnaire – 9 (PHQ-9)	9	Based on criteria for major depressive disorder from DSM including low mood, anhedonia, sleep disturbance, somatic symptoms and suicidal ideation
Anxiety Symptoms		
Generalised Anxiety Disorder-7 (GAD-7)	7	Based on criteria for GAD from DSM including worrying, feeling anxious, restless and irritable
Hospital Anxiety and Depression Scale – Anxiety Subscale (HADS-A)	7	Focused on cognitive symptoms of GAD rather than purely physical symptoms which may reflect condition.

Table 11.1 (continued)

Psychometric tool	N. of Items	Properties assessed
State-Trait Anxiety Inventory (STAI)	40	Evaluates state anxiety (current state of anxiety right now) and trait anxiety (stable aspects of anxiety proneness including calmness, confidence, and security)
Masculinity		
Conformity to Masculine Norms Inventory—Abbreviated	22	Winning, emotional control, risk-taking, violence, dominance, self- reliance, primacy of work, power over women, pursuit of status
Male Role Norms Inventory—Revised	7	Measuring extent to which men feel they can display emotion
Masculinity in Chronic Disease Inventory	28	Strength, sexual importance, family responsibility, emotional self-reliance, optimistic capacity, action approach
Body Image		
Body Image Scale (BIS)	10	Self-consciousness, physical attractiveness, satisfaction with appearance, difficulty seeing self-naked, wholeness of body, dissatisfaction with scars
Concerns About Body Image	3	Loss of muscle, negative feelings about boy look, feelings body is getting soft/flabby
Fear of Cancer Recurrence		
Fear of Cancer Recurrence 7 (FCR7)	7	Measures frequency and severity of fear of developing cancer again along with impact on daily activities/functioning
Cancer Worry Scale (CWS)	8	Evaluates concerns about developing cancer again and impact of these on daily functioning
Fear of Cancer Recurrence Inventory- Short Form (FCRI-SF)	9	Assesses the presence and severity of intrusive thoughts associated with FCR
Self-Esteem		
Rosenberg Self-Esteem Scale	10	Positive and negative statements related to own feelings of self-esteem

Index: *DSM* Diagnostic and Statistical Manual of Mental Disorders, *GAD* Generalised Anxiety Disorder, *FCR* Fear of Cancer Recurrence

Revision Questions

Multiple Choice Questions

1. A 55-year-old male presents with a penile cancer affecting his glans penis. The lymphatics that primarily drain this area are the
   A. Para-aortic lymph nodes
   B. Superficial inguinal lymph nodes
   C. External Iliac Lymph nodes
   D. Deep inguinal Lymph nodes
   E. Para-Caval lymph nodes

2. After bilateral groin node dissection, a patient presents with genital lymphoedema and scarring that does not resolve with elevation, his lymphoedema can be classified as:
   A. Primary
   B. Secondary
   C. Stage 2
   D. Stage 3
   E. Both B & D
3. The most appropriate treatment of a patient with Stage 2, asymptomatic genital lymphoedema would be:
   A. Decongestive lymphatic therapy
   B. Lymph node transfer
   C. Scrotoplasty
   D. Lymphaticovenous anastomosis
   E. Liposuction

Viva Cases

Case 1

A 65-year-old gentleman presents with a mass affecting his glans penis and undergoes a glansectomy and bilateral sentinel node biopsy. Pathology confirms a G3 T2 SCC of the penis and both sentinel nodes contain evidence of metastases.

A. What procedure does he require next?
B. What are the anatomical boundaries of the femoral triangle?
C. What are the potential complications of radical inguinal node dissection?
D. Are there any techniques to reduce the morbidity associated radical lymph node dissection?

   The patient returns after his treatment and has extensive penile and scrotal lymphoedema.

E. How do you manage this complication?

Answers

Multiple Choice Questions

1. **D.** Lymphatics from the penile skin pass to the superficial inguinal nodes whereas the glans penis drains into the deep inguinal lymph nodes.
2. **E.** Lymphoedema post penile cancer treatment is secondary and the staging classification is described in the text. As it does not resolve with elevation it is stage 3.
3. **A.** Decongestive lymphatic therapy includes exercise, compression bandages, diet, elevation and infection prevention

Viva Cases
Case 1

A. Bilateral Radical Inguinal Node Dissection
B. Superiorly – Inguinal ligament
   Lateral – Medial border of Sartorius
   Medial – Lateral border of adductor longus
   Floor – Pectineus muscle/iliopsoas
C. Morbidity can be as high as 50%. Complications include, infection, bleeding, flap necrosis, temporary lymphocele, prolonged lymph drainage and potentially permanent lymphoedema of the genitals and lower limb.
D. Surgical techniques have been adapted and include preservation of the saphenous vein, preservation of the campers and scarpas fascia and more recently the use video endoscopic inguinal lymphadenectomy has shown to be an oncologically safe procedure with lower morbidity, although trials are ongoing.
E. Conservative measures include the use of supportive underwear, exercise and avoidance of trauma to the affected area. Most trusts have a dedicated lymphoedema nurse specialist or team that can treat the patient with Decongestive Lymphatic Therapy (DLT). These treatment strategies include skin care to reduce infection, exercise to assist lymphatic drainage and reduce adipose tissue, and massage and compression techniques to reduce swelling. If the lymphoedema is severe and not responding to these conservative approaches then surgical options include scrotectomy with scrotoplasty and penile unburying, scrotal flaps, skin grafting, tissue debulking or lymphatic restoration at specialist centres.

Test your learning and check your understanding of this book's contents: use the "Springer Nature Flashcards" app to access questions using ▶ https://sn.pub/1r7Om8. To use the app, please follow the instructions in chapter 1.

References

1. Tashiro K, Yamashita S, Saito T, Iida T, Koshima I. Proximal and distal patterns: different spreading patterns of indocyanine green lymphography in secondary lower extremity lymphedema. J Plast Reconstr Aesthet Surg. 2016;69(3):368–75.
2. Zaleska M, Olszewski WL, Durlik M. The effectiveness of intermittent pneumatic compression in long-term therapy of lymphedema of lower limbs. Lymphat Res Biol. 2014;12:103–9.
3. Monteiro LL, Skowronski R, Brimo F, et al. Erectile function after partial penectomy for penile cancer. Int Braz J Urol. 2021;47(3):515–22.
4. Sedigh O, Falcone M, Ceruti C, et al. Sexual function after surgical treatment for penile cancer: which organ-sparing approach gives the best results? Can Urol Assoc J. 2015;9(7–8):E423–7.
5. Preto M, Falcone M, Blecher G, et al. Functional and patient reported outcomes following Total glans resurfacing. J Sex Med. 2021;18(6):1099–103.

6. Sansalone S, Silvani M, Leonardi R, et al. Sexual outcomes after partial penectomy for penile cancer: results from a multi-institutional study. Asian J Androl. 2017;19(1):57–61.
7. Romero FR, Romero KR, Mattos MA, Garcia CR, Fernandes Rde C, Perez MD. Sexual function after partial penectomy for penile cancer. Urology. 2005;66(6):1292–5.
8. Warren AG, Brorson H, Borud LJ, et al. Lymphedema: a comprehensive review. Ann Plast Surg. 2007;59:464–72.
9. Clodius L. Lymphatics, lymphodynamics, lymphedema: an update. Plast Surg Outlook. 1990;4:1.
10. Morey AF, Meng MV, McAninch JW. Skin graft reconstruction of chronic genital lymphedema. Urology. 1997;50:423–6.
11. Namir SA, Trattner A. Transient idiopathic primary penoscrotal edema. Indian J Dermatol. 2013;58(5):408.
12. Smeltzer DM, Stickler GB, Schirger A. Primary lymphedema in children and adolescents: a follow-up study and review. Pediatrics. 1985;76:206.
13. Aulia I, Yessica EC. Surgical management of male genital lymphedema: a systematic review. Arch Plast Surg. 2020;47(1):3–8.
14. Halperin TJ, Salvin SA, Olumi AF, et al. Surgical management of scrotal lymphedema using local flaps. Ann Plast Surg. 2007;59:67–72. discussion 72
15. Modolin M, Mitre AI, da Silva JC, et al. Surgical treatment of lymphedema of the penis and scrotum. Clinics (Sao Paulo). 2006;61:289–94.
16. Bevan-Thomas R, Slaton JW, Pettaway CA. Contemporary morbidity from lymphadenectomy for penile squamous carcinoma: the MD Anderson Cancer Center Experience. J Urol. 2002;167:1638–42.
17. Protzel C, Alcaraz A, Horenblas S, et al. Lymphadenectomy in the surgical management of penile cancer. Eur Urol. 2009;55:1075–88.
18. Alnajjar HM, Castiglione F, Ahmed K, Haider A, Nigam R, Muneer A. A novel 'Batman' scrotectomy technique for the management of scrotal lymphoedema following treatment for penile cancer. Transl Androl Urol. 2019;8(5):448–56.
19. Prostate Cancer UK. Research into wellbeing services for men with prostate cancer –final report 2014 [Available from: https://prostatecanceruk.org/media/2460122/Report-Wellbeing-services-for-men-with-prostate-cancer.pdf.
20. Brunckhorst O, Stewart R, Ahmed K. Ch 20 mind and body in men's health. In: Goonewardene S, Brunckhorst O, Albala D, Ahmed K, editors. Trends in men's health. 1st ed. Springer; 2022.
21. Koch L, Jansen L, Brenner H, Arndt V. Fear of recurrence and disease progression in long-term (>/= 5 years) cancer survivors—a systematic review of quantitative studies. Psychooncology. 2013;22(1):1–11.
22. Cicognani E. Social Well-being. In: Michalos AC, editor. Encyclopedia of quality of life and Well-being research. Dordrecht: Springer Netherlands; 2014. p. 6193–7.
23. Umberson D, Montez JK. Social relationships and health: a flashpoint for health policy. J Health Soc Behav. 2010;51(Suppl):S54–66.
24. Maddineni SB, Lau MM, Sangar VK. Identifying the needs of penile cancer sufferers: a systematic review of the quality of life, psychosexual and psychosocial literature in penile cancer. BMC Urol. 2009;9:8.
25. Paster IC, Chipollini J. Importance of addressing the psychosocial impact of penile cancer on patients and their families. Semin Oncol Nurs. 2022;151286
26. Ficarra V, Righetti R, D'Amico A, Pilloni S, Balzarro M, Schiavone D, et al. General state of health and psychological well-being in patients after surgery for urological malignant neoplasms. Urol Int. 2000;65(3):130–4.
27. Drager DL, Protzel C, Hakenberg OW. Identifying psychosocial distress and stressors using distress-screening instruments in patients with localized and advanced penile cancer. Clin Genitourin Cancer. 2017;15(5):605–9.
28. Harju E, Pakarainen T, Vasarainen H, Tornava M, Helminen M, Perttila I, et al. Health-related quality of life, self-esteem and sexual functioning among patients operated for penile cancer—a cross-sectional study. J Sex Med. 2021;18(9):1524–31.

29. Tornava M, Harju E, Vasarainen H, Pakarainen T, Perttila I, Kaipia A. Men's experiences of the impact of penile cancer surgery on their lives: a qualitative study. Eur J Cancer Care (Engl). 2022;31(1):e13548.
30. Sosnowski R, Wolski JK, Zi Talewicz U, Szyma Ski M, Baku AR, Demkow T. Assessment of selected quality of life domains in patients who have undergone conservative or radical surgical treatment for penile cancer: an observational study. Sex Health. 2019;16(1):32–8.
31. Witty K, Branney P, Evans J, Bullen K, White A, Eardley I. The impact of surgical treatment for penile cancer—patients' perspectives. Eur J Oncol Nurs. 2013;17(5):661–7.
32. Bullen K, Edwards S, Marke V, Matthews S. Looking past the obvious: experiences of altered masculinity in penile cancer. Psychooncology. 2010;19(9):933–40.
33. Yu C, Hequn C, Longfei L, Minfeng C, Zhi C, Feng Z, et al. Sexual function after partial penectomy: a prospectively study from China. Sci Rep. 2016;6:21862.
34. Dinesh AA, Helena Pagani Soares Pinto S, Brunckhorst O, Dasgupta P, Ahmed K. Anxiety, depression and urological cancer outcomes: a systematic review. Urol Oncol. 2021;39(12):816–28.
35. Kiffel J, Sher L. Prevention and management of depression and suicidal behavior in men with prostate cancer. Front Public Health. 2015;3:28.

GPSR Compliance

The European Union's (EU) General Product Safety Regulation (GPSR) is a set of rules that requires consumer products to be safe and our obligations to ensure this.

If you have any concerns about our products, you can contact us on ProductSafety@springernature.com

In case Publisher is established outside the EU, the EU authorized representative is:

Springer Nature Customer Service Center GmbH
Europaplatz 3
69115 Heidelberg, Germany

Batch number: 10372213

Printed by Printforce, the Netherlands